Study Guide for Understanding Medical-Surgical Nursing

SIXTH EDITION

Paula D. Hopper, MSN, RN, CNE
Adjunct Professor
    Spring Arbor University
    Spring Arbor, Michigan
Professor Emeritus
    Jackson College
    Jackson, Michigan

Linda S. Williams, MSN, RN
Master Adjunct Instructor & Professor Emeritus
    Jackson College
    Jackson, Michigan

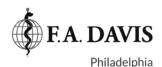

F.A. DAVIS

Philadelphia

F.A. Davis Company
1915 Arch Street
Philadelphia, PA 19103
www.fadavis.com

Printed in the United States of America

Last digit indicates print number: 10 9 8 7 6 5 4 3 2 1

Publisher, Nursing: Terri Wood Allen
Senior Content Project Manager: Elizabeth Hart
Art and Design Manager: Carolyn O'Brien
Digital Project Manager: Sandra Glennie

As new scientific information becomes available through basic and clinical research, recommended treatments and drug therapies undergo changes. The author(s) and publisher have done everything possible to make this book accurate, up to date, and in accord with accepted standards at the time of publication. The author(s), editors, and publisher are not responsible for errors or omissions or for consequences from application of the book, and make no warranty, expressed or implied, in regard to the contents of the book. Any practice described in this book should be applied by the reader in accordance with professional standards of care used in regard to the unique circumstances that may apply in each situation. The reader is advised always to check product information (package inserts) for changes and new information regarding dose and contraindications before administering any drug. Caution is especially urged when using new or infrequently ordered drugs.

ISBN 13: 978-0-8036-6900-0

Preface

NOTE TO THE STUDENT

The *Study Guide for Understanding Medical-Surgical Nursing* has been written and edited exlclusively by us, the authors, to accompany the sixth edition of *Understanding Medical-Surgical Nursing*. We have included exercises that not only help you review content, but also will help you develop your critical thinking abilities. It is essential for you to be able to think critically about the content as you prepare for the NCLEX-PN. We hope you will use this resource as well as Davis Edge and the great resources on Davis Edge.

SUGGESTIONS FOR USING THE STUDY GUIDE

Each chapter includes:

• Case study questions that accompany an audio case study found on Davis Edge. Listen to the scenario and the information noted by both the nurse and the patient to answer the questions.
• An exercise to help you practice chapter vocabulary items. It is important to understand the underlying vocabulary before attempting to apply the terms to understand the remainder of the information in each chapter.
• Basic matching, true/false, word scramble, and other exercises to allow you to practice and understand medical-surgical nursing information. These exercises are most helpful for developing knowledge and recall of material.
• Critical thinking exercises to help you practice your new knowledge in patient situations and make good clinical judgments. We feel strongly that you must learn to think critically, rather than just memorize facts. The answers we provide for the critical thinking exercises are just some of the possibilities. You will come up with additional answers of your own as your knowledge base expands.
• NCLEX-PN–style questions to provide practice in applying your new knowledge. Rationale for why an answer is correct or incorrect has been included to strengthen your critical thinking and test-taking abilities. NEW to the sixth edition: Hot spot questions have been added to some chapters.
• Function and Assessment chapters also include a labeling exercise to help you review basic anatomy.

STUDY GUIDE ANSWERS

• To students: Study Guide answers are posted on the instructor's Davis Edge site. Ask your instructor about accessing answers.
• To instructors: Study Guide answers are posted on the instructor's Davis Edge site. Students do not have access to Study Guide answers. Please provide answers to students according to your needs.

We hope you find this study guide useful. Happy studying and learning to provide safe patient-centered nursing care!

PAULA D. HOPPER AND LINDA S. WILLIAMS

Contents

6   Contents

CHAPTER 1
Critical Thinking and the Nursing Process

Name: _____

Date: _____

Course: _____

Instructor: _____

AUDIO CASE STUDY

Listen to the audio case study available on Davis Edge and then answer the following questions.

Jane and the Nursing Process

1. What are the steps of the nursing process?

   _____

   _____

2. What subjective data did Jane collect about her situation? What subjective data could you collect about your situation as a nursing student trying to balance multiple roles?

   _____

   _____

3. What resources did Jane have to draw on to help her manage the multiple demands on her time? What resources do you have?

   _____

   _____

VOCABULARY

Define the following terms and use them in sentences.

Nursing Process

Definition: _____

_____

Sentence: _____

_____

Critical Thinking

Definition: _____

_____

Sentence: _____

_____

Assessment

Definition: _____

_____

Sentence: _____

_____

Objective Data

Definition: _____

_____

Sentence: _____

_____

Subjective Data

Definition: _____

_____

Sentence: _____

_____

Nursing Diagnosis

Definition: _____

_____

Sentence: _____

_____

Evaluation

Definition: _____

_____

Sentence: _____

_____

Vigilance

Definition: _____

_____

Sentence: _____

_____

SUBJECTIVE AND OBJECTIVE DATA

Identify the following data as subjective (symptom) or objective (sign).

1. Pain _____
2. Shortness of breath _____
3. Edema (swelling) _____
4. Capillary refill 2 seconds _____
5. Nausea _____
6. Vomiting _____
7. Dizziness _____
8. Cyanosis _____
9. Numbness _____
10. Indigestion _____
11. Pale _____
12. Serum potassium 3.6 mEq/L _____
13. Palpitations (feeling of racing heart) _____
14. Blood pressure 130/82 mm Hg _____
15. White blood cell count 7,000/mm^3 _____

CRITICAL THINKING

Sometimes cognitive maps are used to organize thinking. (Look at samples in the aging sections of any of the upcoming function and assessment chapters.) In this workbook, some chapters will ask you to make a cognitive map, so here is an opportunity to practice. Consider a time when you have had a headache or other discomfort. Fill in the spaces with information related to the **WHAT'S UP?** questions. Once you answer the questions, you could go even further and make links with possible interventions. There is no one right way to make a cognitive map—use your imagination!

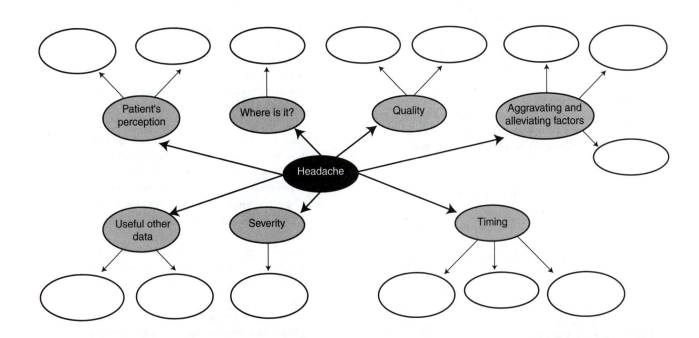

REVIEW QUESTIONS—CONTENT REVIEW

Choose the best answer unless directed otherwise.

1. Which one of the following is a nursing diagnosis?
   1. Peptic ulcer
   2. Pneumonia
   3. Ineffective airway clearance
   4. Myocardial infarction

2. Which one of the following is a medical diagnosis?
   1. Hiatal hernia
   2. Impaired mobility
   3. Powerlessness
   4. Anxiety

3. The nurse is concerned about a piece of unsafe equipment, but the supervisor doesn't feel the concern is important. The nurse approaches the director about the situation. Which critical thinking attitude is the nurse exhibiting?
   1. Intellectual perseverance
   2. Intellectual sense of justice
   3. Intellectual empathy
   4. Intellectual integrity

4. In what order should the nurse carry out the nursing process? Place all steps in correct sequential order.
   1. Implement plan of care.
   2. Assist with evaluation.
   3. Collect data.
   4. Assist with development of nursing diagnoses.
   5. Assist with planning of outcomes and interventions.

5. Which of the following statements best defines *critical thinking*?
   1. Orderly, goal-directed thinking
   2. Clear thinking during critical situations
   3. Constructive feedback about nursing actions
   4. Critical evaluation of patient responses to care

REVIEW QUESTIONS—TEST PREPARATION

Choose the best answer unless directed otherwise.

6. The registered nurse and licensed practical nurse/licensed vocational nurse are reviewing the nursing care plan for a patient with acute pain related to a fractured ankle. Which of the following actions would determine whether the care plan is effective?
   1. Assessment of the patient's ability to walk
   2. Evaluation of the patient's fracture on x-ray
   3. Elevation of the patient's foot on two pillows
   4. Evaluation of the patient's pain rating on a 10-point scale

7. A patient with a history of cardiac disease reports feeling tightness in the chest that radiates down the left arm. Which of the following actions by the licensed practical nurse/licensed vocational nurse should be carried out first?
   1. Check the patient's vital signs.
   2. Formulate nursing diagnoses related to an acute myocardial infarction.
   3. Determine the patient's outcome after nitroglycerin has been administered.
   4. Plan interventions to reduce long-term cardiac damage.

8. The nurse is documenting patient data. Which of the following should the nurse document under objective data? **Select all that apply.**
   1. Coughed up 5 mL yellow sputum
   2. Patient short of breath
   3. Headache in frontal area
   4. Heart rate 72 beats per minute
   5. Hemoglobin level 11.2 g/dL

9. A patient is admitted with chest pain, which has resolved. The patient states, "I hope I can live a normal life." According to Maslow's hierarchy of needs, which of the following levels is best reflected by this statement?
   1. Physiological needs
   2. Safety and security
   3. Love and belonging
   4. Self-esteem

10. A patient has a nursing diagnosis of *Impaired Swallowing* related to muscle weakness as evidenced by drooling, coughing, and choking. Which of the following outcomes is appropriate for this patient's nursing diagnosis?
    1. Improved airway clearance within 8 hours as evidenced by clear lung sounds and productive cough
    2. Baseline body weight maintained as evidenced by no weight loss
    3. Improved muscle strength as evidenced by ability to sit up while eating
    4. Improved swallowing within 48 hours as evidenced by no coughing or choking

11. The nurse is providing care for a patient with a medical diagnosis of congestive heart failure who is very short of breath. Which of the following is a nursing diagnosis that is correctly stated in the PES (problem, etiology, and signs and symptoms) format?
    1. Deficient knowledge related to disease process and self-care for shortness of breath
    2. Impaired gas exchange related to excess interstitial fluid as evidenced by respiratory rate of 32 breaths per minute and patient stating he feels short of breath
    3. Congestive heart failure related to decreased cardiac output as evidenced by abnormal arterial blood gasses
    4. Acute dyspnea related to congestive heart failure as evidenced by swollen lower extremities and confusion

CHAPTER 2
Evidence-Based Practice

Name:	
Date:	
Course:	
Instructor:	

AUDIO CASE STUDY

Listen to the audio case study available on Davis Edge and then answer the following questions.

Marie and Evidence-Based Practice

1. What did Marie learn about thirdhand smoke? Were you aware of thirdhand smoke and the dangers it can pose to patients and others?

2. What is considered the gold standard of health care?

3. What are the six steps in the process of evidence-based practice that Marie and her classmates were using?

4. What did the search reveal is best practice for smoking cessation?

VOCABULARY

Define the following terms.

Evidence-Based Practice
Definition: _____

_____

Sentence: _____

_____

Evidence-Informed Practice
Definition: _____

_____

Sentence: _____

_____

Randomized Controlled Trials
Definition: _____

_____

Sentence: _____

_____

Research
Definition: _____

_____

Sentence: _____

_____

Systematic Review
Definition: _____

_____

Sentence: _____

_____

Health Literacy
Definition: _____

_____

Sentence: _____

_____

EVIDENCE-BASED PRACTICE

1. Evidence is the _____ of effectiveness behind nursing practice.

2. It is important for the _____ in which the evidence will be used to be considered.

3. Evidence-based practice is a complex but important and necessary process to facilitate _____ care and optimal patient outcomes.

4. Evidence-based practice is used by nurses to give the best _____ possible.

5. Level I is the best evidence and is an analysis of many _____ controlled trials.

6. Nurses will know from measured _____ that they are giving the best care possible.

7. Evidence-based practice is considered the

   _____ standard of health care.

8. The Quality and Safety Education for Nurses (QSEN) project focuses on _____ education that promotes the continual improvement of quality and safety in patient care.

9. Patient-centered care meets the needs and preferred schedules.

10. Evidence is the core _____ that directs safe, quality-driven, excellent patient care.

CRITICAL THINKING

Read the following case study and answer the questions.

Nurses on a surgical unit are interested in knowing if music would reduce the preoperative anxiety of patients on their unit.

1. How are these nurses contributing to quality care?

   _____

   _____

2. What should the nurses do to begin the process?

   _____

   _____

3. What are some examples of resources that can be used to find evidence?

   _____

   _____

4. The nurses find Level I research studies that show music therapy can be beneficial in reducing anxiety. What step should the nurses take next?

   _____

   _____

5. The planned intervention is implemented, data are collected during the implementation, and now the pilot study has ended. What step should the nurses take next?

   _____

   _____

REVIEW QUESTIONS—CONTENT REVIEW

Choose the best answer unless directed otherwise.

1. Which of the following is considered significant evidence to guide nursing care?
   1. Research studies that are quasi-experimental
   2. Cochrane Reviews
   3. Nursing information from the Internet
   4. The opinion of a nationally known nursing expert

2. A nurse would like to find other studies on wound care that might be relevant to how wound care is done. Which of the following would be best for searching for nursing articles on wound care?
   1. Cumulative Index to Nursing and Allied Health Literature (CINAHL)
   2. Medline
   3. Cochrane Review
   4. PubMed

3. A nurse on the safety committee is assigned to review the current National Patient Safety Goals. In which of these ways will the nurse find the goals?
   1. Review Joanna Briggs Institute evidence-based resources.
   2. Review a fundamentals nursing textbook.
   3. Go to www.jointcommission.org.
   4. Search Cochrane Reviews.

4. Which of the following best describes a randomized clinical trial?
   1. An observational study designed to collect subjective data
   2. An experimental study in which multiple factors affecting the results are controlled
   3. A specific design categorizing modifiable and nonmodifiable risk factors
   4. Tracking of disease occurrence over a set period of time

5. Evidence-based practice most often begins with which of the following?
   1. Asking how to solve a clinical problem
   2. Initiating a literature search
   3. Analyzing available evidence
   4. Measuring baseline outcomes

REVIEW QUESTIONS—TEST PREPARATION

Choose the best answer unless directed otherwise.

6. The nurse is reviewing the patient's plan of care and ordered treatments. Which of the following is an independent nursing intervention? **Select all that apply.**
   1. Giving acetaminophen (Tylenol) 650 mg orally every 4 hours as needed
   2. Assisting the patient to a position of comfort
   3. Giving hand massages daily
   4. Initiating high-risk fall protocol
   5. Placing the nurse's call button within reach at all times
   6. Teaching deep breathing and relaxation techniques as needed

7. A nurse on the research committee is assigned to review the best evidence on patient-centered bathing. Which of the following kinds of evidence would the nurse select for Level I research? **Select all that apply.**
   1. A Cochrane Review
   2. One randomized controlled trial
   3. Four quasi-experimental studies that show similar results
   4. The opinion of a national nursing expert on the subject
   5. A Joanna Briggs Institute evidence-based resource

8. The nurse will include which of the following in applying the process of evidence-based practice to patient-centered care? **Select all that apply.**
   1. Ask a burning question.
   2. Determine current practice.
   3. Evaluate the change.
   4. Know how to conduct a randomized controlled trial.
   5. Make it happen.
   6. Search for the best available evidence.

9. A nurse is preparing to give oral care to a patient who has halitosis. Which of the following is the best evidence-based method to give oral care? **Select all that apply.**
   1. Use oral foam swabs with water to swab the teeth and mouth.
   2. Use a soft toothbrush and toothpaste to brush the teeth and tongue.
   3. Rinse the mouth with mouthwash after each meal.
   4. Provide breath mints for the patient after each meal.
   5. Floss the teeth daily.

10. A nurse investigating the effect of 12-hour shifts on medication errors identifies 962 articles published on the topic of 12-hour shifts in the past 5 years. Which action should the nurse take next?
    1. Find out how many of the articles can be found at the institution.
    2. Request all 962 articles and determine their validity.
    3. Limit the request to articles published in the past 3 years.
    4. Narrow the search to identify which articles discuss medication errors.

CHAPTER 3
Issues in Nursing Practice

Name:	_____
Date:	_____
Course:	_____
Instructor:	_____

AUDIO CASE STUDY

Listen to the audio case study available on Davis Edge and then answer the following questions.

Jim and the Health Care System

1. What is nursing informatics, the field in which Mario says he is interested in getting an advanced degree?

   _____

   _____

2. What are three examples of nursing interventions to prevent hospital-acquired conditions?

   _____

   _____

3. Why did Jim not provide information to a caller who asked about a patient's condition?

   _____

   _____

VOCABULARY

Match the term with the appropriate definition or statement.

1. _____ Civil law
2. _____ Administrative law
3. _____ Criminal law
4. _____ Administrative policies
5. _____ Mandated reporting law
6. _____ Ethics
7. _____ Nurse practice act
8. _____ Human trafficking
9. _____ Health Insurance Portability and Accountability Act (HIPAA)
10. _____ Liability

1. Laws that license nurses and regulate nursing practice
2. Developed at the organizational level to define an organization's processes for providing care
3. Laws that regulate individual and personal property rights
4. Laws that regulate behaviors within society
5. Systematic approach to understanding an ethical dilemma and examining the best outcome
6. A law that defines the scope of a nurse's practice
7. Act of recruiting, harboring, transporting, providing, or obtaining a person for labor or as a sex worker through force, fraud, or coercion
8. Law that requires nurses to report known or suspected instances of abuse
9. Responsibility for wrongful clinical decisions
10. Law to protect patient information

NURSING PRACTICE AND ETHICAL AND LEGAL PRINCIPLES

1. The health–illness continuum represents the continual shifting between _____-level health and _____ health throughout life.
2. Nurses must be _____ licensed to practice to _____ the public and maintain the _____ of health care services.
3. _____ is the virtue of truthfulness.
4. The ethical principles used when examining bioethical and health care dilemmas include autonomy, _____, nonmaleficence, _____, veracity, and _____.
5. Effective leaders are _____ about the management process, _____ models, positive thinkers, and use _____ to earn the _____ of their coworkers.

VALUES CLARIFICATION

Complete the following sentences.

1. The one thing I have always wanted to do is:

    _____.
    _____.

2. If I inherited $5 million, I would:

    _____.
    _____.

3. As president of the United States, I would:

    _____.
    _____.

4. If I died today, I would like my obituary to say:

    _____.
    _____.

5. If I could control the world and its destiny, I would:

    _____.
    _____.

Complete this list of things people value with any other items you believe should be included, and then rank the value you believe each item has, with 1 being the highest value.

Rank	Valued Item	Rank	Valued Item
_____	Family	_____	Professionalism
_____	Career	_____	_____
_____	Religion	_____	_____
_____	Honor	_____	_____
_____	Material possessions	_____	_____
_____	Health	_____	_____
_____	Recreation	_____	_____

What have you learned about yourself by doing this exercise? What do the rankings signify? Can you identify yourself as more utilitarian or more deontological? (There are no answers to this section because this is an exercise requiring personal responses.)

CRITICAL THINKING

Read the following case study and answer the questions.

Mrs. Reo is a 5 foot, 3 inch, 105-lb, 86-year-old retired cleaning lady. She was admitted to a general medical-surgical unit in a small rural hospital. She was diagnosed 3 months ago with metastatic cancer that has spread from her liver to her lungs and bone marrow. She received chemotherapy and radiation therapy for several weeks, but the treatment was not effective. She was admitted to the hospital because she became too weak to walk or care for herself at home. The cancer returned, and the large doses of oral narcotic medications taken at home were having little effect on her pain while increasing her confusion and weakness.

Her oncologist decided that further chemotherapy or radiation therapy would not be effective, and she ordered Mrs. Reo to be kept comfortable with medications. A continuous morphine intravenous (IV) drip was started to help control the pain. Even with this medication, Mrs. Reo cried out in pain, particularly when morning care was given, and begged the nurses not to move her. Because she was severely underweight, the skin over her bony prominences quickly became reddened and showed the beginning signs of breakdown.

The hospital standards of care for immobile patients require that they be repositioned at least every 2 hours. Mrs. Reo yelled so loudly when she was turned that the nursing staff wondered if they were really helping her or hurting her.

To help decide what should be done, the nurses who provided care to Mrs. Reo called a patient care conference. The manager of the unit stated clearly that the hospital standards of care required Mrs. Reo be repositioned at least every 2 hours to prevent skin breakdown, infections, and perhaps sepsis. In her already weakened condition, an infection or sepsis would most likely be fatal. Betsy, who had been a licensed practical nurse for approximately 15 years, disagreed with the manager. Her feeling was that causing this obviously terminal patient so much pain by turning her was cruel and violated her dignity as a human being. She stated that she could not stand to hear Mrs. Reo yell anymore and refused to take care of her until some other decision was made about her nursing care. Sally, a new graduate nurse, felt that the patient should have some say in her own care and that maybe some type of compromise could be reached about turning her, perhaps turning her less frequently or providing more pain relief medication. Monica, a registered nurse who had worked on the unit for 2 years, felt that the health care provider should make the decision about turning this patient and then the nurses should follow the order. This last suggestion was met with strong negative comments by the other nurses present. They felt that patient comfort and turning were nursing measures.

1. What are the important ethical principles in this dilemma?

   _____

   _____

   _____

2. How does the code of ethics apply to this situation?

   _____

   _____

   _____

3. What are the legal issues?

   _____

   _____

   _____

4. Are there ever any situations in which a nurse might legally and ethically violate a standard of care?

   _____

   _____

   _____

5. What are some other possible solutions to this dilemma? What types of consequences might they have?

   _____

   _____

   _____

(There are no correct answers to this section because this is an ethical exercise that has many choices to be considered for the best outcome for the patient. Discuss your options with classmates.)

REVIEW QUESTIONS—CONTENT REVIEW

Choose the best answer unless directed otherwise.

1. Which of the following ethical principles proposes that the primary goal of health care and nursing is to provide good care for others?
   1. Autonomy
   2. Fidelity
   3. Beneficence
   4. Veracity

2. The ethical principle of nonmaleficence is defined as which of the following?
   1. Health care workers avoiding harm to patients
   2. Telling the truth to patients in all matters
   3. Being faithful to commitments made to patients
   4. The right of self-determination of patients

3. Which of the following is the term used to describe an ethical situation that arises where there is a choice between two equally unfavorable alternatives?
   1. Tort
   2. Ethical antagonism
   3. Contraindication
   4. Ethical dilemma

4. Which of the following is the first step in the ethical decision-making process?
   1. Analyze the alternatives.
   2. Identify the ethical dilemma.
   3. Consider the consequences of the actions.
   4. Make a decision.

5. Ethical dilemmas most often involve which of the following situations?
   1. A conflict of basic human rights
   2. Violations of the nurses' code of ethics
   3. Nurses who do not understand the ethical code
   4. Patients who wish to die

6. When applying the ethical principle of autonomy to patient care, the nurse should understand that which of the following is applicable to autonomy?
   1. Autonomy is an absolute principle that has no exceptions.
   2. Only patients who are awake and oriented have the right to autonomy.
   3. Under certain conditions, autonomy can be limited.
   4. Autonomy is the same as the principle of nonmaleficence.

7. Which of the following punishments distinguishes criminal liability from civil liability?
   1. Personal liability
   2. Financial recovery
   3. Loss of license
   4. Potential loss of freedom

8. Which of the following is an unintentional tort?
   1. Negligence
   2. Outrage
   3. Assault
   4. Privacy invasion

REVIEW QUESTIONS—TEST PREPARATION

Choose the best answer unless directed otherwise.

9. A patient with emphysema is being seen by the home health care nurse. The patient is on oxygen, lives alone, and is able to perform activities of daily living, prepare meals, and do light household tasks with rest periods. The patient is unable to perform yard work, which was a favorite hobby. Which of the following would describe the patient's location on the health–illness continuum?
   1. Near death
   2. High-level wellness
   3. Poor health
   4. Moderate-level wellness

10. A nurses' code of ethics states, "The nurse safeguards the patient's right to privacy by judiciously protecting information of a confidential nature." This statement is based on which of the following principles?
    1. The right to privacy is an inalienable right of all persons.
    2. The nurse–patient relationship is based on trust.
    3. A breach of confidentiality may expose the nurse to liability.
    4. Nurses know what is best for patients' health care.

11. A patient asks the nurse about the purpose of a new medication. The nurse responds, "The medication will help you feel better. Don't worry about it." The nurse's response demonstrates which of the following conditions?
    1. Lack of medication knowledge
    2. Legal obligations
    3. Paternalism
    4. Therapeutic communication

12. The nurse advocates for the best interest of a patient who experienced cardiac arrest and is now unconscious. Which of the following conditions is the most important factor for the nurse to consider?
    1. The patient's wishes as expressed before becoming unconscious
    2. The family's wishes now that the patient can no longer communicate
    3. The patient's chances for survival after the cardiac arrest
    4. The physician's orders regarding future arrest situations

13. The licensed practical nurse/licensed vocation nurse is considering whether the task of taking a blood pressure on a 78-year-old resident with hypertension can be delegated to a nursing assistant. Which of the following steps should the nurse consider in this decision-making process for delegation (see www.ncsbn.org/1625.htm)?
    Select all that apply.
    1. Right task
    2. Right circumstances
    3. Right patient
    4. Right communication
    5. Right supervision
    6. Right route

14. The nurse is assisting with patient data collection in a clinic. The nurse is assigned to a young female patient who has an older male friend present at her bedside. The patient is nervous, timid, very thin, and with poor hygiene and lets the friend answer all the nurse's questions. What actions should the nurse take?
    1. Confront the family friend to allow the patient to answer the questions.
    2. Ask the friend to step out of the room during the examination.
    3. Consult health care team members about suspicions.
    4. Complete data collection.
    5. Whisper to patient she will be saved.
    6. Support calling 911.

CHAPTER 4
Cultural Influences on Nursing Care

AUDIO CASE STUDY

Listen to the audio case study available on Davis Edge and then answer the following questions.

Dan and Cultural Assessment

1. What are some assessment findings that affected Dan's care of Mrs. Basiouny?

   _____

   _____

2. What can happen when cultural background is not considered when caring for a patient?

   _____

   _____

3. How can you develop cultural competence in your practice?

   _____

   _____

VOCABULARY

Match the term with the appropriate definition or statement.

1. _____ Belief
2. _____ Cultural assimilation
3. _____ Cultural awareness
4. _____ Cultural competence
5. _____ Cultural sensitivity
6. _____ Custom
7. _____ Ethnic
8. _____ Ethnocentrism
9. _____ Spirituality
10. _____ Stereotype
11. _____ Value
12. _____ Worldview

1. A usual way of acting in a given situation
2. Accepted as true, need not be proven
3. Focuses on knowledge and appreciation of history and ancestry of other cultures
4. Avoidance of actions that may offend another person's cultural beliefs
5. Belief that "my way is the right way"
6. An opinion or belief about someone because of ethnic background
7. Essence of being and gives purpose to existence
8. Belonging to a subgroup of a larger cultural group
9. Way a person perceives the world
10. The process of taking on a dominant culture's values, sometimes with risk of losing one's own cultural heritage
11. Using knowledge and skills about another culture to provide care
12. A principle or belief that has worth to an individual or group

---

CULTURAL CHARACTERISTICS

Answer the following questions. Discuss with a classmate.

1. What are some examples of primary characteristics of culture?

   _____

   _____

   _____

2. What are some examples of secondary characteristics of culture?

   _____

   _____

   _____

3. What is meant by *traditional health care providers*? Give an example.

   _____

   _____

   _____

4. What are some characteristics of people who are primarily present-oriented? Past-oriented? Future-oriented?

   _____

   _____

   _____

CRITICAL THINKING
Immigrants

There are no correct or incorrect answers to the following question. Share your thoughts with your classmates.

1. Identify health care difficulties that new immigrants must overcome in the United States. How might you, as a nurse, help them overcome these difficulties?

   _____

   _____

   _____

CRITICAL THINKING
Personal Insights

Answer the following questions. Consider how people from other cultures might answer differently. Note: There are no answers to this section because this is an exercise requiring personal responses.

1. What do you personally do to prevent illness?

   _____

   _____

2. What home remedies do you use when you have a minor illness such as a cold or the flu? Do you use over-the-counter medications to treat yourself? How might these over-the-counter medicines cause a problem with prescription medications?

   _____

   _____

   _____

3. What significance does food have to you besides satisfying hunger?

   _____

   _____

   _____

4. Are you usually on time for social events? For appointments? Why or why not?

   _____

   _____

   _____

5. Consider what gives your own life hope, meaning, and purpose, and what informs your personal values. Write down the guiding principles of your life.

   _____

   _____

   _____

CRITICAL THINKING
Bathing

Read the following case study and answer the questions. Note: There are no answers to this section because this is an exercise requiring personal responses.

An older adult male patient refuses to be bathed by a female nurse's aide. He has not been bathed for 3 days, and today he really needs a bath. His family is at his bedside.

1. Why might he be refusing his bath?

   _____

   _____

2. What alternatives do you have?

   _____

   _____

3. What is the best solution to the problem?

   _____

   _____

REVIEW QUESTIONS—CONTENT REVIEW

Choose the best answer unless directed otherwise.

1. Patients of Eastern European Jewish heritage should be provided information on which disorder?
   1. Sickle cell anemia
   2. Thalassemia
   3. Lactose intolerance
   4. Tay-Sachs disease

2. A patient states, "I don't know why that foreign doctor needs to be here. I only want to see American doctors." This is an example of which of the following principles?
   1. Cultural sensitivity
   2. Cultural diversity
   3. Ethnocentrism
   4. Acculturation

3. Hispanic Americans and American Indians generally have a _____ glucose level than whites.
   1. Higher
   2. Lower

REVIEW QUESTIONS—TEST PREPARATION

Choose the best answer unless directed otherwise.

4. A 12-year-old child whose family recently immigrated to the United States is newly diagnosed with diabetes mellitus. The home health care nurse is to teach the patient and family diabetes care. Both parents and the child can administer his insulin and recite the signs and symptoms of hypoglycemia and hyperglycemia. They are highly educated and read and speak English well. Which is the best first step in teaching them about nutrition therapy for diabetes?
   1. Give them a food exchange list for a diabetic diet.
   2. Determine whether they can calculate carbohydrates in a sample meal.
   3. Assess current dietary food practices.
   4. Have them make an appointment with a consulting dietitian.

5. A 46-year-old patient has been admitted for breast cancer. The patient wants a religious counselor to visit. Which action should the nurse take?
   1. Ask the nursing supervisor to see if a visit from a religious counselor is permitted.
   2. Tell the patient that religious counselors are not permitted in the hospital.
   3. Suggest that the patient see a hospital priest instead.
   4. Tell the patient a visit is fine, but for safety reasons the patient should tell the nurse or physician before accepting any treatments.

6. An elderly patient is in the operating room having cardiac surgery. In the patient's culture, extended family is highly valued. Eighteen family members arrive on the unit and wait in the patient's room, which is shared by two other patients. Which is the best solution to this problem?
   1. Allow two family members to wait in the room and send the rest of them to the cafeteria.
   2. Send all of them to the lobby and tell them they will be notified when the patient returns to the room.
   3. Allow only the patient's husband and mother to visit.
   4. Assign the patient to a private room and allow the family to wait there.

7. A 42-year-old patient is 40 pounds overweight. Food traditionally enjoyed in this patient's culture is typically high in fat. Indeed, the patient admits to baking pies with lard and frying food in bacon grease, practices the patient does not wish to stop. To reduce fat and calories, what can the home health care nurse encourage the patient to do?
   1. Stop purchasing lard.
   2. Reduce the portion size when cutting the pies.
   3. Bake two separate pies, one for the patient and one for family.
   4. Continue baking with lard but reduce calories from other foods in the patient's diet.

8. A 41-year-old woman has had a mastectomy in the treatment for breast cancer. The belief that God has power over illness is common in this patient's culture. Her physician recommends radiation therapy. She says, "What is the use? My life is in God's hands anyway." Which of the following responses is appropriate?
   1. Agree with the patient but tell her she must accept the radiation or she will die.
   2. Ensure that the patient understands all the implications of the decision before accepting it.
   3. Keep encouraging the patient to think about the radiation, and ask other staff to do the same.
   4. Have the patient ask the physician to prescribe chemotherapy instead of radiation therapy.

9. A 72-year-old patient refuses to take a morning antibiotic, which is scheduled every 8 hours, because the patient is celebrating Ramadan and desires to fast from sunup to sundown. Which of the following actions should the nurse take?
   1. Explain that the medicine must be taken now to maintain the blood level of the drug.
   2. Rearrange the medication schedule so the patient can take all his medicines between sundown and sunup.
   3. Omit the medicine and record the patient's refusal on the medication administration record.
   4. Ask the patient's family to encourage the patient to take the medicine.

10. A 38-year-old female is admitted with ovarian cancer and is receiving her first dose of chemotherapy. She says, "I don't understand how this could happen to me. I'm only 38 and have two children. How am I supposed to deal with this?" Which of the following responses demonstrates patient-centered spiritually effective care?
    1. Ask the patient to complete a religious preference questionnaire to assess her spirituality.
    2. Share personal belief that everything happens for a reason and that the patient will eventually understand.
    3. Ask the patient what has helped in the past that might help coping now with this disease.
    4. Ask why the patient feels she must deal with this alone and recommend calling someone for help.

CHAPTER 5
Complementary and Alternative Modalities

Name:	
Date:	
Course:	
Instructor:	

AUDIO CASE STUDY

Listen to the audio case study available on Davis Edge and then answer the following questions.

Susan and Complementary Therapy

1. What is the difference between complementary and alternative modalities?

   _____

   _____

2. What techniques helped Susan get over her fear of needles?

   _____

   _____

3. What precautions should you teach patients to take when trying new therapies?

   _____

   _____

VOCABULARY

Match the term with the appropriate definition or statement.

1. _____ Alternative modality
2. _____ Complementary modality
3. _____ Homeopathy
4. _____ Naturopathy
5. _____ Ayurvedic
6. _____ Chiropractic

1. Illness is a result of falling out of balance with nature
2. Uses nutrition, herbs, and hydrotherapy
3. Illness is a result of nerve dysfunction
4. Added to a conventional therapy
5. Unconventional therapy
6. "Like cures like"

COMPLEMENTARY MODALITY: GUIDED IMAGERY

Describe the purpose of guided imagery. Write a teaching plan on how to do guided imagery. Try teaching it to a family member or friend.

Purpose: _____

_____

_____

Teaching Plan: _____

_____

_____

_____

CRITICAL THINKING

Read the following case study and answer the questions.

Mrs. Lawless is admitted to your unit with heart failure and fluid overload. As you collect admission data, you find that she is taking feverfew, capsaicin, and St. John's wort regularly in addition to prescribed medications for heart failure. When you question her, she says that the salesperson at the health food store told her these herbs were safe to use with her other medications.

1. What is feverfew used for? _____

_____

_____

2. What is capsaicin used for? _____

_____

_____

3. What is St. John's wort used for? _____

_____

_____

4. Where can you get information about the safety of taking these herbs if the patient has heart failure or is taking heart failure medications? _____

_____

_____

5. What should you tell Mrs. Lawless? _____

_____

_____

REVIEW QUESTIONS—CONTENT REVIEW

Choose the best answer unless directed otherwise.

1. Which of the following therapies would be considered a complementary modality?
   1. Using inhalers in addition to oral medications for asthma
   2. Participating in a cardiac rehabilitation program after having a heart attack
   3. Using echinacea instead of antibiotics for an upper respiratory infection
   4. Using progressive muscle relaxation in addition to muscle relaxants for back pain

2. Which of the following therapies would be considered an alternative modality?
   1. Using hydrotherapy in place of nonsteroidal anti-inflammatory drugs for arthritis
   2. Visiting a spiritual healer in addition to receiving chemotherapy for cancer treatment
   3. Using antibiotics and bronchodilators for acute bronchitis
   4. Using aspirin for a headache

3. Which of the following terms describes traditional Western medicine?
   1. Homeopathy
   2. Naturopathy
   3. Allopathy
   4. Ayurveda

4. Which of the following herbal remedies is possibly effective against viruses and colds?
   1. Echinacea
   2. Feverfew
   3. Chamomile
   4. Ginger

5. The nurse recognizes which of the following as complementary or alternative modalities aimed at altering the body's energy? **Select all that apply.**
   1. Reiki
   2. Magnet therapy
   3. Music therapy
   4. Hydrotherapy
   5. Yoga
   6. Therapeutic touch

REVIEW QUESTIONS—TEST PREPARATION

Choose the best answer unless directed otherwise.

6. The nurse has provided instruction to a patient on how to use guided imagery. Which of the following statements by the patient would indicate to the nurse that further teaching is required?
   1. "I will focus on my breathing."
   2. "I imagine the ocean, including the smell, the sound, and the feel of the air."
   3. "I will relax all parts of my body."
   4. "I will keep my eyes open until the exercise is complete."

7. A patient tells a nurse that a chiropractor is going to do minor surgery to remove a small superficial lump on the patient's neck. Which response by the nurse is best?
   1. "The lump is likely pressing against a nerve; that is why it needs to be removed."
   2. "You need to question your chiropractor's qualifications. Chiropractors do not perform surgery."
   3. "Chiropractors specialize in nerve function. Removing the lump will restore normal nerve function."
   4. "Surgery might not be necessary. Usually a simple chiropractic adjustment will relieve pressure on a nerve."

8. A patient admitted with chronic pain is interested in pursuing an alternative modality for pain but is unsure how to determine whether it is safe. Which of the following responses by the nurse is best?
   1. "As long as the therapy does not include medication, it should be safe."
   2. "You should talk with your health care provider before trying anything new."
   3. "Be careful, because many alternative modalities have dangerous side effects."
   4. "Traditional analgesics are always the safest treatment for chronic pain."

9. A nurse is interested in providing therapeutic touch for a home health care patient with severe pain. This will be the nurse's first experience with therapeutic touch. Which of the following steps is least appropriate to take before providing this new service?
   1. Obtain permission from the patient's health care provider and the home health care agency.
   2. Take classes on how to administer therapeutic touch.
   3. Tell the patient he will be able to reduce the number of medications he takes.
   4. Read current research on the use of therapeutic touch.

10. A patient is preparing to go home from the hospital after an anterior wall myocardial infarction. The patient has new prescriptions for isosorbide mononitrate (Imdur), warfarin (Coumadin), atorvastatin (Lipitor), and aspirin. The patient also takes metformin (Glucophage) and glipizide (Glucotrol XL) for type 2 diabetes and takes self-prescribed ginseng daily. Which initial response by the nurse is best?
   1. "Ginseng can effectively lower blood glucose in patients with diabetes. It is a good choice for you."
   2. "Ginseng is a relatively safe herbal agent. Be sure to check out a reliable website for interactions before continuing to take it at home."
   3. "Ginseng, like other herbal agents, is unsafe to take with your prescribed medications."
   4. "I am concerned that ginseng could interact with your prescribed medications and affect your blood glucose and your blood clotting."

CHAPTER 6
Nursing Care of Patients With Fluid, Electrolyte, and Acid–Base Imbalances

Name:	
Date:	
Course:	
Instructor:	

AUDIO CASE STUDY

Listen to the audio case study available on Davis Edge and then answer the following questions.

Grandma Lois Is Dehydrated

1. What signs of dehydration did Jon find in his grandma?

   _____

   _____

2. What signs of fluid overload did she develop?

   _____

   _____

3. Why are older patients at higher risk for fluid imbalances?

   _____

   _____

VOCABULARY

Fill in the blanks with key terms from the chapter.

1. The process through which a solute moves from an area of higher to an area of lower concentration is

_____.

2. A fluid that has the same osmolarity as blood is said to be _____.

3. A fluid that has a higher osmolarity than blood is said to be _____.

4. A decrease in blood volume is called _____.

5. Electrolytes in the blood that have a positive charge are called _____.

6. The patient with an excess of sodium in the blood has _____.

7. The patient with not enough potassium in the blood has _____.

8. The patient with not enough calcium in the blood has _____.

9. _____ occurs when the serum pH falls below 7.35.

10. If the serum pH is too high, the condition is called _____.

DEHYDRATION

Circle the errors in the following paragraph and write in the correct information.

Mrs. White is a 78-year-old woman admitted to the hospital with a diagnosis of severe dehydration. The licensed practical nurse/licensed vocational nurse (LPN/LVN) assigned to Mrs. White is asked to collect data related to fluid status. The LPN/LVN expects Mrs. White's blood pressure to be elevated because of fluid loss. The nurse also finds Mrs. White's skin turgor to be taut and firm, and notes that the urine output is copius and dark amber. The nurse asks Mrs. White if she knows where she is and what day it is, because severe dehydration may cause confusion. In addition, the nurse initiates intake and output measurements because this is the most accurate way to monitor fluid balance.

ELECTROLYTE IMBALANCES

Match the electrolyte imbalance with its signs and symptoms.

1. _____ Hyponatremia
2. _____ Hyperkalemia
3. _____ Hypokalemia
4. _____ Hypercalcemia
5. _____ Hypocalcemia

1. Osteoporosis, hyperactive reflexes
2. Muscle weakness, weak pulse
3. Muscle weakness, kidney stones
4. Fluid balance, mental status changes
5. Muscle cramps, irregular heart rate

CRITICAL THINKING

Read the following case study and answer the questions.

Mr. James is an 89-year-old man admitted to your unit with worsening chronic bronchitis. On admission, he is short of breath, but he is able to walk to the bathroom without difficulty. The physician orders bronchodilators, antibiotics, and an intravenous (IV) infusion of normal saline at 150 mL per hour. When you return to work the next day, you find Mr. James gasping for breath, coughing, and panicky. You quickly listen to his lungs and hear more moist crackles than you did yesterday.

1. What additional data do you collect to confirm your suspicion of fluid overload?

_____

_____

_____

_____

2. You report your findings to the registered nurse (RN) and collaborate on quickly developing a nursing diagnosis of excess fluid volume. What factors contributed to this problem?

_____

_____

_____

_____

3. The RN pages the health care provider while you return to check on the patient. What nursing interventions can help until orders are received?

_____

_____

_____

_____

4. How will you know when the problem has been resolved?

_____

_____

_____

_____

REVIEW QUESTIONS—CONTENT REVIEW

Choose the best answer unless directed otherwise.

1. Which of the following intravenous solutions is hypotonic?
   1. Normal saline
   2. 0.45% saline
   3. Ringer's lactate
   4. 5% dextrose in normal saline

2. Which of the following hormones retains water in the body?
   1. Antidiuretic hormone
   2. Thyroid hormone
   3. Adenosine triphosphate
   4. Insulin

3. Which food should be avoided by the patient on a low-sodium diet?
   1. Applesauce
   2. Deli turkey
   3. Chicken
   4. Broccoli

4. Which food is recommended for the patient who must increase intake of potassium?
   1. Bread
   2. Eggs
   3. Potatoes
   4. Cereal

5. Which is the most reliable method for monitoring fluid balance?
   1. Daily intake and output
   2. Daily weight
   3. Vital signs
   4. Skin turgor

6. An older adult patient presents to the emergency department reporting severe vomiting and diarrhea, sweating, and rapid heartbeat but has a normal temperature. In continuing the assessment of the patient, what should the nurse first suspect?
   1. Hypervolemia
   2. Dehydration
   3. Edema
   4. Hyponatremia

REVIEW QUESTIONS—TEST PREPARATION

Choose the best answer unless directed otherwise.

7. Which patient is most at risk for fluid volume overload?
   1. The 40-year-old with meningitis
   2. The 35-year-old with kidney failure
   3. The 60-year-old with psoriasis
   4. The 2-year-old with influenza

8. Which patients should be monitored closely for dehydration? **Select all that apply.**
   1. A 50-year-old with an ileostomy
   2. A 19-year-old with chronic asthma
   3. A 22-year-old with diabetes mellitus
   4. A 45-year-old with a temperature of 102.3°F
   5. A 28-year-old with a broken femur
   6. A 36-year-old taking diuretic therapy

9. An older-adult nursing home resident who has always been alert and oriented is now showing signs of dehydration and has become confused. Which electrolyte imbalance is most likely involved?
   1. Hyponatremia
   2. Hyperkalemia
   3. Hypercalcemia
   4. Hypomagnesemia

10. The nurse is caring for a patient with osteoporosis who appears weak and frail. Which of the following nursing interventions is best?
    1. Maintain bed rest.
    2. Encourage fluids.
    3. Ambulate with assistance.
    4. Provide a high-protein diet.

11. A 19-year-old patient develops symptoms of respiratory alkalosis related to an anxiety attack. Which nursing intervention is most appropriate?
    1. Make sure the patient's oxygen is being administered as ordered.
    2. Have patient breathe into a paper bag.
    3. Place patient in a semi-Fowler position.
    4. Have patient do coughing and deep-breathing exercises.

12. A patient has chronic respiratory acidosis related to long-standing lung disease. Which of the following problems is the cause?
    1. Hyperventilation
    2. Hypoventilation
    3. Loss of acid by kidneys
    4. Loss of base by kidneys

13. The nurse is providing discharge instructions for a patient taking an oral potassium chloride supplement. Which of the following statements by the patient indicates that more teaching is needed? **Select all that apply.**
    1. "I won't use salt substitutes that have potassium until I talk to my doctor."
    2. "I need to have my blood checked routinely."
    3. "I should take my supplement first thing in the morning and then wait 30 minutes before eating."
    4. "If the pill is too big to swallow, I can crush it."
    5. "I should call the doctor if I have nausea, vomiting, or abdominal cramps."
    6. "I can expect some diarrhea with this medication."

CHAPTER 7

Nursing Care of Patients Receiving Intravenous Therapy

Name:	_____
Date:	_____
Course:	_____
Instructor:	_____

AUDIO CASE STUDY

Listen to the audio case study available on Davis Edge and then answer the following questions.

Mrs. Andrews's Complications of IV Therapy

1. What equipment should you gather to start intravenous (IV) therapy? (See "Initiating Peripheral Intravenous Therapy" under Procedures on Davis*Plus*.)

   _____

   _____

2. Why did Polly choose to use the indirect method for inserting the cannula?

   _____

   _____

3. Why was an electronic infusion device important for Mrs. Andrews?

   _____

   _____

4. How did Polly know that Mrs. Andrews was developing fluid overload?

   _____

   _____

VOCABULARY

Match the term with the appropriate definition or statement.

1. _____ Intravenous	1. Inside a vein
2. _____ Cannula	2. Seepage of IV fluid into tissues
3. _____ Distal	3. Nearest to the point of attachment or the trunk
4. _____ Infiltration	4. Inflammation of a vein
5. _____ Peripherally inserted central catheter	5. Access device inserted into a superficial peripheral vein and advanced into the central system to the superior vena cava
6. _____ Hematoma	6. An IV needle or catheter with a stylet
7. _____ Phlebitis	7. Farthest from the center or from the trunk
8. _____ Proximal	8. A localized collection of blood in the subcutaneous tissue from a break in a blood vessel

COMPLICATIONS OF IV THERAPY

Fill in the blank with the correct complication.

1. Pain and inflammation at the IV insertion site is called

   _____.

2. Redness and exudate at the IV insertion site indicate the presence of _____.

3. Infiltration into tissue by an IV fluid or drug is called

   _____.

4. Dyspnea and crackles can be a sign of

   _____.

5. A cool, puffy insertion site indicates

   _____.

6. Fever, chills, and tachycardia indicate a systemic infection called _____.

7. Sharp pain at the IV site during infusion of a cold fluid indicates a _____.

8. If the patient develops cyanosis, hypotension, and loss of consciousness, the nurse should suspect

   _____.

CRITICAL THINKING

Read the following case study and answer the questions.

Mr. Livesay is admitted with cellulitis and is receiving IV fluids by gravity drip. When you check his IV, you find it is not dripping.

1. What data can you collect to determine the cause of the problem?

   _____

   _____

   _____

2. What is the role of the licensed practical nurse/licensed vocational nurse?

   _____

   _____

   _____

3. When must the registered nurse be consulted?

   _____

   _____

   _____

   _____

CALCULATION PRACTICE

Calculate the answers to the following problems. Round each answer to the nearest whole number.

1. June has an IV of 5% dextrose in water ordered to infuse at 83 mL/hr. How many drops per minute should be set if the tubing delivers 15 drops per mL?

   _____

2. Frank has a piggyback antibiotic of 500 mg in 50 mL of 5% dextrose in water. The medication must infuse over 20 minutes. The tubing drip factor is 10. How many drops per minute? _____

3. Dave has an IV of normal saline ordered at 1 L over 12 hours. How many mL per hour should he receive?

   _____

4. Lucy has an order to administer 800 units of heparin per hour. The registered nurse hangs heparin 50,000 units in 500 mL of 5% dextrose in water. It will run on an electronic infusion device. How many mL should be administered per hour? _____

5. Jack has an order for 1,000 mL of normal saline over 24 hours. How many drops should be administered per minute, using microdrop tubing? _____

REVIEW QUESTIONS—CONTENT REVIEW

Choose the best answer unless directed otherwise.

1. Which of the following complications can occur if a clotted cannula is aggressively flushed?
   1. A clot can enter the circulation.
   2. An air embolism can enter the circulation.
   3. A painful arterial spasm can occur.
   4. The patient can experience speed shock.

2. Which of the following symptoms most likely indicates that an infusion is infiltrated?
   1. Redness at the site
   2. Pain at the site
   3. Puffiness at the site
   4. Exudate at the site

3. An 87-year-old patient recovering from abdominal surgery has a continuous intravenous infusion to supply nutrients and antibiotics. What complication should you suspect when signs and symptoms of redness, warmth, and pain at the infusion site are reported?
   1. Phlebitis
   2. Thrombosis
   3. Hematoma
   4. Infiltration

4. A patient in an outpatient oncology clinic is going to have a peripherally inserted central catheter line placed and wants to know what that means. What is the best response by the nurse?
   1. "It is a catheter that is inserted into your jugular vein and ends in the central circulation."
   2. "It is just a regular IV, but an extra-small catheter is used to prevent vein irritation."
   3. "It is a percutaneous intravenous core catheter."
   4. "It is an intravenous device that is inserted into your arm and ends in the circulation near your heart."

REVIEW QUESTIONS—TEST PREPARATION

Choose the best answer unless directed otherwise.

5. Which patient would benefit most from a capped intravenous access that is used intermittently rather than continuously?
   1. The patient with pneumonia who needs fluids and antibiotics
   2. The patient who has had major blood loss after a motor vehicle accident
   3. The young child who is dehydrated
   4. The older patient who is receiving a diuretic for fluid overload

6. The physician orders furosemide (Lasix) 40 mg intravenous push STAT for a patient in acute fluid overload. Why was the intravenous route likely chosen?
   1. Furosemide can be administered only by the intravenous route.
   2. Intravenous push is the route of choice for rapid action.
   3. Intravenous push dosing is more accurate.
   4. Intravenous push furosemide has fewer side effects than oral.

7. A patient has orders to receive 1 L (1,000 mL) of 5% dextrose and lactated Ringer solution to be infused over 8 hours. How many mL will be infused per hour?
   1. 80
   2. 100
   3. 125
   4. 150

8. A patient is receiving an intravenous piggyback antibiotic in 50 mL of 5% dextrose in water to run over 1 hour. The tubing has a drop factor of 60. How many drops per minute should be delivered?
   1. 6
   2. 17
   3. 50
   4. 100

9. A patient is receiving an intravenous solution delivered by an electronic control device. The alarm sounds, and the display panel indicates occlusion. The nurse pushes the alarm silence button, but the alarm quickly resumes. Which of the following actions should be taken first?
   1. Notify the health care provider.
   2. Check for kinking of the tubing or a closed clamp.
   3. Turn off the intravenous solution, and gently flush the line with 3 mL of saline solution.
   4. Decrease the rate to 10 mL/hr, and flush the line with 1 mL of heparin solution.

CHAPTER 8
Nursing Care of Patients With Infections

Name: _____

Date: _____

Course: _____

Instructor: _____

AUDIO CASE STUDY

Listen to the audio case study available on Davis Edge and then answer the following questions.

Tisha and Treating Patients With Infections

1. What are characteristics of methicillin-resistant *Staphylococcus aureus* (MRSA)?

   _____

   _____

2. What are standard precautions?

   _____

   _____

3. How can vancomycin-resistant *Enterococci* (VRE) be transmitted?

   _____

   _____

4. What does Tisha do after her shift ends to protect herself and prevent transmitting infectious organisms to her home?

   _____

   _____

VOCABULARY

Define the following terms and use them in a sentence.

Antigen

Definition: _____

_____

Sentence: _____

_____

Asepsis

Definition: _____

_____

Sentence: _____

_____

Bacteria

Definition: _____

_____

Sentence: _____

_____

Clostridium Difficile (C. diff)

Definition: _____

_____

Sentence: _____

_____

Hand hygiene

Definition: _____

_____

Sentence: _____

_____

Pathogens

Definition: _____

_____

Sentence: _____

_____

Personal Protective Equipment

Definition: _____

_____

Sentence: _____

_____

Phagocytosis

Definition: _____

_____

Sentence: _____

_____

Sepsis

Definition: _____

_____

Sentence: _____

_____

Virulence

Definition: _____

_____

Sentence: _____

_____

Viruses

Definition: _____

_____

Sentence: _____

_____

PATHOGEN TRANSMISSION

Match the pathogen with its mode of transmission.

1. _____ Zika virus disease   1. Vehicle-borne
2. _____ Malaria   2. Droplet
3. _____ Tuberculosis   3. Airborne
4. _____ Rocky Mountain   4. Vector-borne
            spotted fever
5. _____ Meningitis
6. _____ Pneumonia
7. _____ Measles
8. _____ Influenza
9. _____ Pneumonic plague
10. _____ Hepatitis A

PATHOGENS AND INFECTIOUS DISEASES

Fill in the blanks with the appropriate pathogen or infectious disease name.

1. _____ Gram-positive bacteria clusters that can cause pneumonia, cellulitis, peritonitis, and toxic shock.

2. _____ Group of plantlike organisms that includes yeast and molds; rarely pathogenic.

3. _____ A fungus that can cause thrush.

4. _____ The virus that causes infectious mononucleosis.

5. _____ A systemic fungal respiratory disease caused by *Histoplasma capsulatum.*

6. _____ A disease caused by infection with the protozoan *Toxoplasma gondii.*

7. _____ Single-celled parasitic organisms that move and live mainly in the soil.

8. _____ Small intracellular parasites that can live only inside cells; may produce disease when they enter a cell.

9. _____ A bacterium that must be inside living cells to reproduce and cause disease; causes Rocky Mountain spotted fever.

10. _____ Bleach is used to kill its spores.

CRITICAL THINKING

Read the following case study and answer the questions.

A 72-year-old patient is admitted to a private room with an antibiotic-resistant respiratory tract infection.

1. What equipment is needed for transmission-based precautions?_____

_____

_____

_____

2. What type of equipment would be used for collecting patient data and nursing interventions?

_____

_____

_____

3. Describe the psychosocial effects on a patient in isolation.

_____

_____

_____

4. What can you include in the plan of care for a patient in isolation to reduce social isolation?

_____

_____

_____

5. What condition is the patient at risk of developing during antibiotic treatment for this infection?

_____

_____

_____

REVIEW QUESTIONS—CONTENT REVIEW

Choose the best answer unless directed otherwise.

1. Which of the following would the nurse recognize as a sign of a local infection during data collection?
   1. Warm skin
   2. Clammy skin
   3. Anorexia
   4. Pale nailbeds

2. Which of the following does the nurse understand is a sterile technique?
   1. Use of antiseptics
   2. Use of autoclaves
   3. Frequent hand washing
   4. Use of gloves when coming in contact with body fluids

3. Which of the following infections would the nurse recognize as being a health care–associated infection?
   1. Chronic urinary tract infection for a homebound person
   2. A sexually transmitted infection in a healthy young adult
   3. Pneumonia in a hospitalized postoperative patient
   4. A person with diabetes who requires hospitalization for cellulitis

4. Which of the following antibiotics would the nurse anticipate would be used to treat methicillin-resistant *Staphylococcus aureus* (MRSA)?
   1. Gentamicin
   2. Tobramycin
   3. Penicillin
   4. Vancomycin

5. Which of the following does the nurse understand is needed by all pathogenic organisms to multiply? **Select all that apply.**
   1. Moisture
   2. Light
   3. Food
   4. Oxygen
   5. Warmth

REVIEW QUESTIONS—TEST PREPARATION

Choose the best answer unless directed otherwise.

6. Which of the following actions would be appropriate for the nurse to take while providing patient care to help prevent the spread of organisms? **Select all that apply.**
   1. Sterilizing hands with a germicide once a day
   2. Cleaning stethoscope before and after each patient use.
   3. Performing hand hygiene before and after each patient contact
   4. Wearing gloves for all patient care
   5. Assisting patient with hand hygiene after toileting
   6. Offering patient disinfecting wipes before meals

7. In planning care for a patient, the nurse understands that surgical asepsis is based on which of the following principles?
   1. Destroying organisms before they enter the body
   2. Isolating all patients who have infectious diseases
   3. Destroying bacteria as they leave the body
   4. Maintaining basic cleanliness

8. A nurse must apply a fit-tested high-efficiency particulate air (HEPA) filter mask when entering the room of a patient with which of these infections?
   1. Influenza
   2. Scabies
   3. Human immunodeficiency virus (HIV)
   4. Tuberculosis

9. The nurse is to collect a sterile urine specimen. Which of these actions should the nurse use in collecting this specimen? **Select all that apply.**
   1. Cleansing the patient's external genitalia before the patient voids
   2. Having the patient void into a sterile container
   3. Straight catheterizing the patient
   4. Obtaining a midstream voided specimen
   5. Obtaining a second voiding specimen
   6. Placing catheterized urine specimen in a sterile container

10. Which of the following actions can the nurse take to help prevent a health care–associated infection in an incontinent patient?
    1. Avoiding use of a urinary catheter
    2. Applying absorbent briefs
    3. Toileting patient every 4 hours
    4. Restricting fluids

11. A patient has been diagnosed recently as having an upper respiratory infection. Which of the following symptoms would indicate to the nurse that the patient is developing a complication?
    1. Scratchy throat
    2. Clear, watery drainage from the nose
    3. Dry cough
    4. Temperature 103°F (39.4°C)

12. The nurse is collecting a culture of wound drainage, and the patient asks what a culture is. Which of the following is the best response by the nurse to explain what a culture is?
    1. "A culture identifies the presence of pathogens."
    2. "A culture measures antibiotic levels."
    3. "A culture identifies an antibiotic's effect on a pathogen."
    4. "A culture determines the appropriate medication dosage."

13. Which of the following data collection findings should the nurse recognize and report as a possible sign of infection in the older adult? **Select all that apply.**
    1. Poor skin turgor
    2. Irritability
    3. Hypertension
    4. Restlessness
    5. Pacing behavior
    6. Hunger

14. The nurse observes a nursing assistant providing oral care to an immunocompromised patient. The use of which of the following by the nursing assistant would require further instruction for patient safety?
    1. Sterile water
    2. Tap water
    3. Fluoride toothpaste
    4. Soft toothbrush

15. The nurse is responding to the call light of a patient who has tuberculosis. Mark the area where the nurse would wear the most essential personal protective equipment prior to entering the room of this patient.

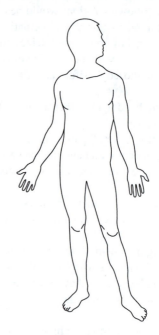

CHAPTER 9
Nursing Care of Patients in Shock

Name:	
Date:	
Course:	
Instructor:	

AUDIO CASE STUDY

Listen to the audio case study available on Davis Edge and then answer the following questions.

José and Anaphylactic Shock

1. What is the correct way to remove an insect stinger from the skin? Did José perform this task correctly?

   _____

   _____

2. Why did Anna ask about prior bee stings?

   _____

   _____

3. Why is it important to teach José to have an epinephrine autoinjector with him at all times?

   _____

   _____

VOCABULARY

Fill in the blank with the word formed by word building.

1. _____ acid (sour) + osis (condition)
2. _____ an- (without) + aerobic (presence of oxygen)
3. _____ an- (without) + phylaxis (protection)
4. _____ a (without) + rhythmia (rhythm)
5. _____ cardia (heart) + genesis (beginning)
6. _____ cyan (blue coloring) + osis (condition)
7. _____ tachy (fast) + pnea (breathing)
8. _____ olig (few) + uria (urine)
9. _____ tachy (fast) + cardia (heart)
10. _____ hypo (low) + perfuser (to pour over or through)

MATCHING

Match the area of the cardiovascular system that contributes to the development of shock with each type of shock.

1. _____ Hypovolemic shock   1. Heart
2. _____ Cardiogenic shock   2. Blood vessels
3. _____ Anaphylactic shock   3. Fluid volume
4. _____ Septic shock
5. _____ Neurogenic shock

SIGNS AND SYMPTOMS OF SHOCK STAGES

Fill in the blank lines to complete the table.

Signs/Symptoms	Stages		
	Compensated	**Progressive**	**Irreversible**
Heart rate	Tachycardia	_____	Slowing
Pulses	_____	Weak, thready	_____
Systolic blood pressure	Normal	Below 90 mm Hg In hypertensive person, 25% below baseline	_____
Diastolic blood pressure	_____	_____	Decreasing to 0
Respirations	_____, deep	Tachypnea, crackles, _____	_____, irregular, shallow
Temperature	Varies	Decreased, can rise in septic shock	_____
Level of consciousness	_____ _____ Sense of impending doom	Confused, lethargic	Unconscious, comatose
Skin and mucous membranes	Cool, clammy, pale	Moist, cold, clammy, pale	_____ _____ _____ Clammy
Urine output	_____	_____	15 mL/hr decreasing to anuria
Bowel sounds	_____	Decreasing	_____

CRITICAL THINKING

Identify the stage of shock, category of shock, and initial action to take for the following patients.

1. An 80-year-old woman admitted with a bowel obstruction has minimal urine output. A nasogastric tube has 1,500 mL of bloody aspirate returned on insertion. She becomes comatose. Vital signs are as follows: blood pressure 78 mm Hg with Doppler stethoscope, pulse 140 bpm and thready, respiration rate 8 breaths per minute, and temperature 94°F (34°C).
   Stage: _____
   Category of Shock: _____
   Initial Action: _____

2. A 56-year-old patient with chronic kidney disease who receives hemodialysis is agitated. Her blood pressure is 100/92 mm Hg, pulse 110 bpm, respiration rate 18 breaths per minute, and temperature 102°F (39°C).
   Stage: _____
   Category of Shock: _____
   Initial Action: _____

3. A 50-year-old patient who is hypotensive is receiving a fluid challenge of 1,000 mL 0.9% normal saline over 4 hours. Her lung sounds are now crackles in all lung fields. Her heart rhythm is irregular. Jugular vein distention and ankle edema are present. Blood pressure has dropped from 96/50 to 80/40 mm Hg in 1 hour, pulse 108 bpm, respiration rate 24 breaths per minute, and temperature 95°F (35°C). She is confused.
   Stage: _____
   Category of Shock: _____
   Initial Action: _____

REVIEW QUESTIONS—CONTENT REVIEW

Choose the best answer unless directed otherwise.

1. Which of the following actions would the nurse take to collect data to determine status of peripheral tissue perfusion in a 48-year-old patient in shock?
   1. Obtain apical pulse.
   2. Check capillary refill.
   3. Check for sacral edema.
   4. Monitor level of consciousness.

2. Which of the following does the nurse understand is the primary reason that respiration increases in compensated shock?
   1. Anxiety causes hyperventilation.
   2. Retention of carbon dioxide is decreased.
   3. Normal oxygen levels are maintained.
   4. Cardiac output is increased.

3. With which of the following stages of shock would the nurse anticipate the skin to be cold and moist during data collection?
   1. Compensated
   2. Progressive
   3. Irreversible

4. The nurse is caring for a hypertensive patient whose blood pressure is usually 156/86 mm Hg. Which of the following blood pressures is considered a progressive shock blood pressure finding for this patient?
   1. 90/44 mm Hg
   2. 140/80 mm Hg
   3. 114/64 mm Hg
   4. 130/72 mm Hg

5. Which of the following outcomes for the nursing diagnosis *Deficient Knowledge* is appropriate for the patient recovering from shock?
   1. Accepts responsibility for shock
   2. States understanding of shock
   3. Interacts with others
   4. Verbalizes fears

REVIEW QUESTIONS—TEST PREPARATION

Choose the best answer unless directed otherwise.

6. The nurse monitors a patient with chronic kidney disease who has just completed a hemodialysis session. The patient's data before dialysis was as follows: blood pressure 150/88 mm Hg, pulse 90 bpm, respiration rate 18 breaths per minute, temperature 98.9°F (37°C), and weight 168 pounds. Patient data obtained after dialysis is as follows: blood pressure 98/50 mm Hg, pulse 110 bpm, respiration rate 18 per minute, temperature 99°F (37°C), and weight 165 pounds. Which of the following actions should the nurse take after comparing the data?
   1. Reweigh the patient.
   2. Provide a quiet environment so the patient may rest.
   3. Notify the health care provider of the postdialysis data.
   4. Monitor the patient in 10 minutes.

7. A 47-year-old patient is admitted with hypovolemic shock from trauma injuries resulting from an automobile accident. The patient remains oliguric 2 days later. Which of the following assessments of the patient indicates to the nurse that the patient is experiencing a complication of shock that requires follow-up treatment?
   1. Hematocrit 42% (normal = 38% to 47%)
   2. Creatinine 2.2 mg/dL (normal = 0.6 to 1.3 mg/dL)
   3. Blood urea nitrogen 24 mg/dL (normal = 6 to 25 mg/dL)
   4. Hemoglobin 13.4 g/dL (normal = 13.5 to 18 g/dL)

8. The nurse is caring for a patient with a bowel obstruction. Which of the following is the earliest indication that the patient is developing symptoms of shock?
   1. Blood pressure 88/50 mm Hg
   2. Pulse 110 bpm
   3. Lethargy
   4. Urine 18 mL/hr

9. The nurse is caring for a postoperative patient following a splenectomy. Which of the following symptoms is of highest priority for the nurse to report?
   1. Blood pressure 86/52 mm Hg
   2. Pulse 100 bpm
   3. Cool, pale skin
   4. Urine 40 mL/hr

10. The nurse is caring for a patient with gastrointestinal bleeding who has an intravenous infusion of 0.9% normal saline at 50 mL/hr. The patient has a large, red, bloody stool and reports dizziness. The nurse assists the patient back to bed and obtains the following vital signs: blood pressure 90/52 mm Hg, pulse 118 bpm, and respiration rate 22 per minute. Which of the following actions should the nurse take?
    1. Continue monitoring vital signs.
    2. Inform the registered nurse now.
    3. Decrease the intravenous fluid flow rate.
    4. Elevate the head of the bed.

11. Which of the following medications would the nurse anticipate the health care provider may order to increase blood pressure for a patient with septic shock?
    1. Atropine
    2. Digoxin
    3. Nitroglycerin
    4. Norepinephrine

12. For the patient in hypovolemic shock, place the following interventions in the order of priority in which the nurse should perform them.
    1. Record hourly urine output.
    2. Apply oxygen.
    3. Provide restful environment.
    4. Ensure patent airway.
    5. Obtain vital signs.
    6. Monitor prescribed intravenous fluids.

13. The nurse is providing care for a patient with pericardial effusion who is at risk for pericardial tamponade. Which of the following symptoms would indicate the patient is developing obstructive shock? **Select all that apply.**
    1. Blood pressure 88/56 mm Hg
    2. Urine output 100 mL over 6 hours
    3. Pulse 66 bpm
    4. Respirations 12 per minute
    5. Jugular vein distention
    6. Confusion and lethargy

14. The nurse is providing care to a patient experiencing shock and should be vigilant for signs of which of the following complications that are related to prolonged shock? **Select all that apply.**
    1. Acute respiratory distress syndrome
    2. Cystic fibrosis
    3. Disseminated intravascular coagulation
    4. Multiple organ dysfunction syndrome
    5. Polycythemia vera
    6. Sickle cell anemia

CHAPTER 10
Nursing Care of Patients in Pain

Name:	_____
Date:	_____
Course:	_____
Instructor:	_____

AUDIO CASE STUDY

Listen to the audio case study available on Davis Edge and then answer the following questions.

Wilma Gets a Lesson in Pain Control

1. Wilma had an episode of acute pain. What is the difference between acute and chronic pain?

   _____

   _____

2. What are the components of a good pain assessment?

   _____

   _____

3. What nursing precautions should be taken when administering opioids? Nonsteroidal anti-inflammatory drugs (NSAIDs)?

   _____

   _____

4. Why might NSAIDs be more effective than opioids for an acute injury like Wilma's?

   _____

   _____

VOCABULARY

Match the term with the appropriate definition or statement.

1. _____ Addiction
2. _____ Tolerance
3. _____ Ceiling effect
4. _____ Pain
5. _____ Prostaglandins
6. _____ Adjuvant
7. _____ Opioid
8. _____ Patient-controlled analgesia
9. _____ Endorphins
10. _____ Analgesic

1. Whatever the experiencing person says it is
2. Endogenous chemicals that act like opioids
3. Larger dose of analgesic required to relieve same pain
4. Psychological dependence
5. Self-administered analgesics
6. Dose of analgesic limited by side effects
7. Medication that relieves pain
8. Drug used to potentiate analgesics
9. Neurotransmitters released during pain
10. A morphinelike drug

CULTURALLY RESPONSIVE CARE

1. Mrs. Walker, a new patient on your unit, has recently been admitted for rehabilitation following a hip fracture. She has a son who is very engaged in her care. He visits his mother several times a week and will often bring a small bottle of oil with him that he will dab on his finger and then use to make the sign of the cross on her forehead. What is the best response?
   1. Ask the son about the oil and other family beliefs that are important in healing.
   2. Ask the son to refrain from using any substances on the patient's skin without approval from the doctor.
   3. Document what you saw and continue passing medications.
   4. Instruct the nursing assistants to go to the room and watch what else he does.

2. How might you further engage Mrs. Walker's son in her care?
   _____
   _____

3. When you go to check on Mrs. Walker a few hours later, you notice that she is frowning, her teeth are clenched tight, and she is wringing her hands. You ask her if she is having any pain, and she responds, "No." How do you respond?
   1. Say, "Okay" and document that the patient currently has no reported pain.
   2. Advise the patient that it is time for her next scheduled pain medication and go retrieve it.
   3. Tell the patient that you noticed her frowning and clenching her teeth, and ask if her hip is sore or if she is uncomfortable.
   4. Call the patient's son and ask him to talk to her about being honest about her pain.

CRITICAL THINKING

Read the following case study and answer the questions.

Ms. Murphy is a 32-year-old woman admitted to your unit following an emergency appendectomy at 0800. When you enter her room at 1400, she is sitting up in bed smiling and visiting with her family. She tells you she is hurting and asks for her pain medication. You check her medication record and find orders for morphine 5 to 10 mg intravenous push every 4 hours as needed for pain.

1. List at least seven areas you will assess related to her pain. _____
   _____
   _____
   _____

2. Based on your assessment, you discuss administering 10 mg of morphine with the registered nurse, who will give the intravenous medication. What class of drugs does morphine belong to? What is its mechanism of action? Why is it important for you to be aware of these things when the registered nurse is administering the drug? _____
   _____
   _____
   _____

3. What is the most effective medication schedule that can be implemented today? _____

_____

_____

_____

4. What side effects will you watch for? _____

_____

_____

_____

5. How will you know if the medication has been effective?

_____

_____

_____

_____

6. The next morning you decide to administer Tylenol #3 (acetaminophen 300 mg with codeine 30 mg) for Ms. Murphy's pain, but it is not effective. Why do you think it did not help? _____

_____

_____

_____

_____

7. What nondrug therapies might be appropriate for Ms. Murphy? What technique has already been effective for her? _____

_____

_____

_____

_____

REVIEW QUESTIONS—CONTENT REVIEW

Choose the best answer unless directed otherwise.

1. Which of the following definitions of pain is most appropriate to use when planning nursing care?
   1. Knife-like sensation along a nerve pathway
   2. Burning sensation that accompanies severe injury or trauma
   3. Injured tissues responding with release of neuro-transmitters that cause a sensation of pressure or discomfort
   4. Whatever the experiencing person says it is, occurring whenever the person experiencing it says it does

2. Which of the following terms describes a feeling of threat to one's self-image or life that may accompany pain?
   1. Fear
   2. Anxiety
   3. Suffering
   4. Panic

3. Which of the following is a common side effect of opioid administration?
   1. Constipation
   2. Respiratory depression
   3. Tachycardia
   4. Addiction

4. Which of the following is the most accurate way to assess the severity of a patient's pain?
   1. Observe for moaning or other physical signs.
   2. Watch for elevated blood pressure and pulse.
   3. Have the patient rate pain on a standard pain scale.
   4. Monitor the frequency with which the patient requests pain medication.

5. Which of the following statements best explains why a patient can be laughing and talking and yet still be in pain?
   1. Most patients try to deny their pain because pain is socially unacceptable.
   2. Distraction can help relieve pain when used in combination with analgesics.
   3. Most patients who are laughing and talking are not in pain.
   4. Laughing prolongs the effects of opioids in the body.

REVIEW QUESTIONS—TEST PREPARATION

Choose the best answer unless directed otherwise.

6. An 82-year-old patient in a long-term care facility has been receiving intramuscular meperidine (Demerol) for chronic back pain. After several weeks, the patient becomes irritable, which is a change from normal behavior. Which response by the nurse is best?
   1. Understand that chronic pain can cause a patient to become irritable.
   2. Obtain an order for an adjuvant sedative to administer with the meperidine.
   3. Request a psychiatric referral to evaluate the patient's mental status.
   4. Consult with the registered nurse or health care provider about changing to a different analgesic.

7. A nurse is caring for a patient who reports being in severe pain. The patient has an order for hydrocodone/acetaminophen (Norco) 2 tabs every 6 hours as needed for pain. Before providing the medication, which of the following actions should the nurse take?
   1. Verify the patient's liver and kidney function studies are within normal limits.
   2. Determine the patient's current pulse rate and blood glucose level.
   3. Assess the patient's pain level and respiratory rate.
   4. Identify the emotional or physical cause of the patient's pain.

8. A patient with severe pain is receiving narcotic pain medication via a patient-controlled analgesia pump. The nurse notes that the patient is lethargic and difficult to arouse with a respiratory rate of 7 breaths per minute. After informing the registered nurse, which of the following drugs does the nurse anticipate will be ordered?
   1. Naloxone (Narcan)
   2. Methadone (Dolophine)
   3. Hydrocodone/acetaminophen (Norco)
   4. Phenytoin (Dilantin)

9. A patient has chronic pain for which no cause can be found. The health care provider orders a placebo. Which response by the nurse to the health care provider is best?
   1. "I will give the placebo and document the patient's response."
   2. "I know if the placebo helps the pain, then the pain is not real."
   3. "I am not comfortable administering this placebo without the patient's consent."
   4. "May we alternate the placebo with an opioid order?"

10. A patient has a patient-controlled analgesia pump following spinal surgery. The patient appears to be in pain but is too drowsy to push the button on the pump. Which response by the nurse is correct?
    1. Push the button for the patient.
    2. Instruct the patient's family member to push the button, not to exceed every 10 minutes.
    3. Assess the patient's vital signs.
    4. Increase the dose of medication delivered in each injection.

11. A patient with a known history of cocaine abuse is admitted after a motorcycle accident. The patient calls you into the room and says, "I need something for this pain. Now." Which assumption by the nurse is best?
    1. The patient is withdrawing from cocaine and needs an opioid to reduce symptoms.
    2. The patient is in pain and needs an analgesic.
    3. The patient is trying to establish control over the situation.
    4. The patient is faking pain to gain access to opioids.

12. The nurse is providing care for a patient in the emergency department who is experiencing a migraine headache. The patient reports taking two extra-strength acetaminophen (Tylenol) 500 mg tablets every 6 hours for the past few days. The nurse would be most concerned by which of the following statements by the patient?
    1. "I usually drink three or four beers a day."
    2. "My headache pain is six out of ten."
    3. "I'm having difficulty sleeping."
    4. "It hurts even worse with these bright lights."

CHAPTER 11
Nursing Care of Patients With Cancer

Name:	
Date:	
Course:	
Instructor:	

AUDIO CASE STUDY

Listen to the audio case study available on Davis Edge and then answer the following questions.

Michael Manages Side Effects of Chemotherapy

1. What symptoms should you be vigilant for during the nadir following chemotherapy?

_____

_____

2. Why are patients short of breath when they are anemic?

_____

_____

3. Why did Michael grab the apple off Mr. Woo's lunch tray?

_____

_____

VOCABULARY

Fill in the blank.

1. Loss of hair is called _____.

2. Loss of appetite is called _____.

3. _____ places the patient at risk of infection.

4. Dry mouth is called _____.

5. Treatment aimed at maintaining comfort is called _____ therapy.

6. _____ is the use of drugs to combat cancer.

7. Substances that poison cells are described as _____.

8. _____ is the term used to describe a new growth.

9. When cancer _____, it travels to a new site.

10. A tumor that is not cancerous is called _____.

11. A _____ is done to obtain a tissue sample to detect cancer cells.

12. Agents that prevent damage to healthy cells from chemotherapy or radiation are called _____ agents.

CELLS

Label each statement as true or false and correct the false statement.

1. _____ Chromosomes are made of DNA and protein.

2. _____ A gene is the code for one DNA molecule.

3. _____ Messenger RNA carries the genetic code to the cell membrane.

4. _____ A genetic change in a cell is called a *mutation*.

5. _____ Transfer RNA brings amino acids to the proper sites on the DNA.

6. _____ Cells become malignant by mutating.

7. _____ In any human cell, most of the genes are always active.

8. _____ The chromosome number for a human cell is 48.

9. _____ The process of mitosis produces two identical cells with 23 chromosomes each.

10. _____ Mitosis is necessary only for growth of the body.

BENIGN VERSUS MALIGNANT TUMORS

Compare the characteristics of benign and malignant tumors. List as many characteristics as you can remember.

_____

_____

_____

_____

_____

CRITICAL THINKING

Delmae is a 48-year-old restaurant worker undergoing chemotherapy following a right modified mastectomy. List two or three nursing interventions for each of the side effects she can expect to experience.

1. Leukopenia: _____

_____

_____

_____

2. Thrombocytopenia: _____

_____

_____

3. Anemia: _____

_____

_____

4. Stomatitis: _____

_____

_____

5. Nausea and vomiting: _____

_____

_____

6. Alopecia: _____

_____

_____

REVIEW QUESTIONS—CONTENT REVIEW

Choose the best answer unless directed otherwise.

1. Genes are made of which of the following?
   1. Chromosomes
   2. Deoxyribonucleic acid
   3. Ribonucleic acid
   4. Protein

2. Which is the correct term used for a group of similar cells found on an external or internal body surface?
   1. Skin
   2. Mucous membrane
   3. Epithelial tissue
   4. Connective tissue

3. Which of the following foods can increase cancer risk?
   1. Broccoli, cauliflower
   2. Butter, ice cream
   3. Chicken, fish
   4. Cakes, breads

4. A nurse is caring for a patient with a radioactive implant. How can the nurse avoid unnecessary radiation exposure?
   1. Avoid entering the patient's room more than once every 24 hours.
   2. Limit the amount of time spent with the patient.
   3. Avoid touching the patient.
   4. Place a "contaminated" sign on the patient's bed.

REVIEW QUESTIONS—TEST PREPARATION

Choose the best answer unless directed otherwise.

5. A patient is admitted with suspected lung cancer and asks, "How will my physician know for sure if I have cancer?" Which of the following responses is correct?
   1. "Your physician will do cultures of your sputum."
   2. "An x-ray examination will be done to confirm the diagnosis."
   3. "A biopsy is the only way to know for sure."
   4. "Your physician will do a bronchoscopy to view the cancer."

6. Which of the following nursing interventions will help relieve symptoms of mucositis related to radiation therapy?
   1. Provide frequent mouth care.
   2. Offer cold liquids often.
   3. Provide high-carbohydrate foods.
   4. Offer juices frequently.

7. A patient is receiving chemotherapy after surgery for prostate cancer. Which of the following signs or symptoms indicates that the patient is experiencing thrombocytopenia?
   1. Fever
   2. Petechiae
   3. Pain
   4. Vomiting

8. How can the nurse best prevent complications in the patient with leukopenia? **Select all that apply.**
   1. Wash hands frequently.
   2. Avoid injections.
   3. Allow no visitors.
   4. Provide colony-stimulating factors as ordered.
   5. Monitor temperature every 4 hours.
   6. Offer fresh fruits and vegetables.

9. A patient has severe pain related to bone cancer. The nurse notes that the patient does not ask for pain medication while watching television. Which of the following statements best explains this?
   1. Distraction is a good pain relief method and can prevent the need for analgesics.
   2. The patient may ask for pain medication when the television is not on because of boredom.
   3. The pain must be psychosomatic because it is relieved by television.
   4. Distraction can be a helpful intervention when used in addition to analgesics.

10. A patient with terminal cancer is referred to hospice for support. How can hospice help the patient and family? **Select all that apply.**
    1. Hospice nurses can help administer curative chemotherapy.
    2. Hospice supports research efforts in finding cancer cures.
    3. Hospice can help the patient's family keep the patient comfortable until death.
    4. Hospice can help the patient find financial resources for cancer treatment.
    5. Hospice can provide follow-up counseling after the patient's death.
    6. Hospice can provide respite care for family members or caregivers.

11. The nurse is providing care for a patient in an outpatient surgical center anticipating a needle biopsy of suspicious nodules in the left lung. The patient asks, "If they think this might be cancer, why don't they just cut it all out?" Which of the following responses by the nurse is best?
    1. "Most patients who have lung biopsies don't end up having cancer."
    2. "Why do they think you have cancer?"
    3. "The biopsy will determine if you have cancer and, if so, what treatment is best."
    4. "It does seem odd that the doctor didn't simply schedule surgery."

CHAPTER 12
Nursing Care of Patients Having Surgery

Name: _____	
Date: _____	
Course: _____	
Instructor: _____	

AUDIO CASE STUDY

Listen to the audio case study available on Davis Edge and then answer the following questions.

Alan and the Surgical Patient

1. What items on the surgical checklist are completed or verified to prepare the patient for surgery?

   _____

   _____

   _____

2. What does Alan do to the patient's bed upon Mrs. Spring's return to her room after surgery?

   _____

   _____

   _____

3. What are some things Alan does to promote patient safety for Mrs. Spring after surgery?

   _____

   _____

   _____

4. What exercises did Alan help Mrs. Spring perform to prevent complications?

   _____

   _____

   _____

VOCABULARY

Fill in the blank.

1. _____ are physicians who perform surgical procedures.

2. The three surgical phases are referred to collectively by the term _____.

3. The _____ phase begins with the decision to have surgery and ends with transfer of the patient to the operating room.

4. The _____ phase begins when the patient is transferred to the operating room and ends when the patient is admitted to the perianesthesia care unit (PACU).

5. The _____ phase begins with the admission of the patient to the PACU and continues until the patient's recovery is completed.

6. _____ is the period when an anesthetic is first given until full anesthesia is reached.

7. An _____ agent is a medication (such as narcotics, muscle relaxants, or antiemetics) used with the primary anesthetic agents.

8. The sudden bursting open of a wound's edges that may be preceded by an increase in serosanguineous drainage is referred to as _____.

9. _____ are physicians who administer anesthesia.

10. _____ causes a loss of sensation and allows the surgical procedure to be done safely.

11. _____ occurs from hypoventilation or mucous obstruction that prevents some alveoli from opening and being fully ventilated.

12. _____ is the removal of necrotic and infected tissue.

13. _____ is a body temperature that is below normal range.

14. _____ is the viscera spilling out of the abdomen.

15. A _____ is an advance practice registered nurse certified to provide anesthetics to surgical patients.

SURGERY URGENCY LEVELS

Match the surgery urgency level to the appropriate definition or example. The level may be used more than once.

1. _____ Surgery needed when any delay jeopardizes the patient's life or limb

2. _____ Fracture repair

3. _____ Surgery needed within 24 to 30 hours

4. _____ Extremity emboli

5. _____ Surgery planned and scheduled without immediate time constraints

6. _____ Surgery done at request of the patient

7. _____ Hernia repair

8. _____ Rhinoplasty

9. _____ Infected gallbladder

10. _____ Cosmetic surgery

1. Optional
2. Elective
3. Urgent
4. Emergency

NOURISHING THE SURGICAL PATIENT

Find the seven errors and insert the correct information.

Healing requires increased vitamin A for collagen formation, vitamin B_{12} for blood clotting, and magnesium for tissue growth, skin integrity, and cell-mediated immunity. Carbohydrates are essential for controlling fluid balance and manufacturing antibodies and white blood cells. Hypoalbuminemia, a low urine albumin, impedes the return of interstitial fluid to the venous return system, decreasing the risk of shock. A serum zinc level is a useful measure of protein status.

COMPLICATION PREVENTION

Indicate whether the statement is true or false and correct the false statement.

1. _____ All medications that patients are taking must be reviewed preoperatively.
2. _____ Most anticoagulants, such as warfarin (Coumadin), do not need to be stopped before surgery.
3. _____ Patients with diabetes who take insulin may be told to take half of their normal insulin dose on the day of surgery.
4. _____ One method to prevent wrong site surgery is for the nurse to mark the site before surgery begins.
5. _____ If a patient is on chronic oral steroid therapy, the steroid therapy cannot be abruptly stopped when the patient is nil per os (NPO; nothing by mouth).
6. _____ Blood glucose monitoring for patients who are diabetic is ordered on admission to the surgical unit.
7. _____ Chronic oral steroid therapy should be continued via the parenteral route if the patient is NPO.
8. _____ Circulatory collapse can develop if steroids are not stopped abruptly.
9. _____ Indwelling urinary catheters are not a source of infection for a surgical patient.
10. _____ Intermittent pneumatic compression devices can cause blood clots.

PERIOPERATIVE NURSING DIAGNOSES AND OUTCOMES

Write a patient objective (goal) for each nursing diagnosis.

Preoperative

1. *Anxiety* or *Fear* related to potential change in body image, hospitalization, pain, loss of control, and uncertainties surrounding surgery

   _____

   _____

2. *Deficient Knowledge* related to lack of previous experience with surgical routines and procedures

   _____

   _____

Intraoperative

3. *Risk for Injury* related to perioperative positioning, chemicals, electrical equipment, and effect of being anesthetized

   _____

   _____

4. *Risk for Impaired Skin Integrity* related to chemicals, positioning, and immobility

   _____

   _____

Postoperative

5. *Acute Pain* related to tissue damage from surgery, muscle spasms, nausea, or vomiting

   _____

   _____

6. *Risk for Infection* related to inadequate primary defenses from surgical wound

   _____

   _____

WOUND HEALING PHASES

Complete the table.

Phase	Time Frame	Wound Healing	Patient Effect
Phase I	_____		Fever, malaise
Phase II	_____	Granulation tissue forms	_____
Phase III	_____	Collagen deposited	_____
Phase IV	Months to 1 year	_____	_____

CRITICAL THINKING

Read the case study and answer the questions.

Mrs. Vell, age 74, is scheduled for a total hip replacement because of osteoarthritis. She is seen in the preadmission testing department 2 weeks before surgery.

1. Why is Mrs. Vell being seen in preadmission testing?

   _____

   _____

   _____

2. What preadmission testing may be done?

   _____

   _____

   _____

3. What teaching should the nurse do in preadmission testing?

   _____

   _____

   _____

   _____

   _____

   _____

4. What are the responsibilities of the admitting nurse to prepare Mrs. Vell for surgery?

   _____

   _____

   _____

   _____

5. What is the role of the holding area nurse?

   _____

   _____

   _____

   _____

   _____

6. What is a role of the licensed practical nurse/licensed vocational nurse in the operating room?

   _____

   _____

   _____

7. What are the two prioritized primary responsibilities of the perianesthesia care nurse?

   _____

   _____

8. Explain why postoperative care for this patient includes pain control, deep breathing and coughing, leg exercises, activity, and leg abduction.

   _____

   _____

   _____

   _____

REVIEW QUESTIONS—CONTENT REVIEW

Choose the best answer unless directed otherwise.

1. Which of the following is a licensed practical nurse/
   licensed vocational nurse patient care role in the
   preoperative phase?
   1. Obtaining preoperative orders
   2. Explaining the surgical procedure
   3. Offering emotional support
   4. Providing informed consent

2. When the patient's signature is witnessed by the nurse
   on the surgical consent, which of the following does the
   nurse's signature indicate?
   1. The nurse obtained informed consent.
   2. The nurse provided informed consent.
   3. The nurse answered all surgical procedure questions.
   4. The nurse verified that the patient signed the consent.

3. Which of the following is an intraoperative outcome for
   a patient undergoing an inguinal hernia repair?
   1. Verbalizes fears.
   2. Maintains skin integrity.
   3. Demonstrates leg exercises.
   4. Explains deep-breathing exercises.

4. Which of the following is a discharge criterion from the
   perianesthesia care unit for a patient after surgery?
   1. Oxygen saturation is above 90%.
   2. Oxygen saturation is below 90%.
   3. The patient has voided.
   4. Intravenous narcotics have been given less than
      30 minutes earlier.

5. Which of the following are discharge criteria from ambulatory surgery that would allow the patient to be discharged following surgery? **Select all that apply.**
   1. Is able to drive self home
   2. Has a landline home telephone
   3. Understands discharge instructions
   4. Has received intravenous narcotics 20 minutes prior
   5. Will be released to a responsible adult
   6. Plans to rest for 24 hours

REVIEW QUESTIONS—TEST PREPARATION

Choose the best answer unless directed otherwise.

6. The nurse is caring for a patient in the preoperative
   period who, even after verbalizing concerns and having
   questions answered, states, "I know I am not going to
   wake up after surgery." Which of the following actions
   should the nurse take?
   1. Reassure the patient everything will be all right.
   2. Inform the registered nurse.
   3. Explain the national surgery death rate.
   4. Ask family to comfort the patient.

7. The nurse understands that which of the following is the
   reason that long-term steroid therapy cannot be abruptly
   stopped? **Select all that apply.**
   1. Higher steroid levels are needed during stress.
   2. Malignant hyperthermia will result.
   3. Hypertensive crisis will occur.
   4. Respiratory failure will occur.
   5. Circulatory collapse may result.

8. The nurse is to provide preoperative teaching for a
   74-year-old patient. Which of the following actions
   should the nurse take to improve learning? **Select all
   that apply.**
   1. Allow patient increased time to respond.
   2. Determine readiness to learn.
   3. Present one idea at a time.
   4. Speak in a high tone.
   5. Use blue and green color brochures.
   6. Use medical terminology.

9. The nurse is teaching a postoperative patient about
   complications. Which of the following would the nurse
   explain might be prevented with early postoperative
   ambulation? **Select all that apply.**
   1. Increased peristalsis
   2. Coughing
   3. Pneumonia
   4. Evisceration
   5. Deep vein thrombosis
   6. Paralytic ileus

10. Which of the following actions should the nurse take to maintain patient safety when ambulating a patient for the first time postoperatively?
    1. Use one person to assist the patient.
    2. Use two people to assist the patient.
    3. Encourage the patient to stand quickly.
    4. Give narcotic 15 minutes before ambulation.

11. The nurse is caring for a patient with a bowel resection. Which of the following would indicate that the patient's gastrointestinal tract is resuming normal function?
    1. Firm abdomen
    2. Excessive thirst
    3. Presence of flatus
    4. Absent bowel sounds

12. The patient is sitting at the bedside and states, "Oh, my stomach is tearing open." Which of the following actions is a priority for the nurse to take when dehiscence occurs?
    1. Have patient sit upright in a chair.
    2. Decrease rate of intravenous fluids.
    3. Have patient lie down.
    4. Obtain a sterile suture set.

13. The nurse is assisting the patient to use an incentive spirometer. Which of the following actions by the patient indicates that the patient needs further teaching on how to use the spirometer?
    1. Taking two normal breaths before use
    2. Inhaling deeply to reach target
    3. Sitting upright before use
    4. Exhaling to reach target

14. After surgery, the nurse notes that the patient's urine is dark amber and concentrated. Which of the following does the nurse understand may be the reason for this?
    1. The sympathetic nervous system saves fluid in response to stress of surgery.
    2. The sympathetic nervous system diureses fluid in response to stress of surgery.
    3. The parasympathetic nervous system saves fluid in response to stress of surgery.
    4. The parasympathetic nervous system diureses fluid in response to stress of surgery.

15. The patient develops a low-grade fever 18 hours postoperatively and has diminished breath sounds. Which of the following actions is most appropriate for the nurse to take to prevent complications? **Select all that apply.**
    1. Administer antibiotics.
    2. Encourage coughing and deep breathing.
    3. Administer acetaminophen (Tylenol).
    4. Decrease fluid intake.
    5. Ambulate patient as ordered.
    6. Monitor output.

16. The nurse explains how to use an incentive spirometer to a patient who is to have surgery. Mark the area where the incentive spirometer will help prevent atelectasis postoperatively.

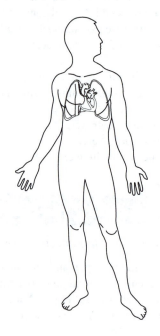

CHAPTER 13
Nursing Care of Patients With Emergent Conditions and Disaster/Bioterrorism Response

Name: _____

Date: _____

Course: _____

Instructor: _____

AUDIO CASE STUDY

Listen to the audio case study available on Davis Edge and then answer the following questions.

Tabitha and the Emergency Department

1. What is the purpose of using cervical spine, or C-spine, precautions in a trauma patient?

   _____

   _____

2. What did Tabitha see as effects of cardiac tamponade in one of her patients?

   _____

   _____

3. What was the significance of the steering wheel damage and the patient's report of tenderness in the middle of his chest?

   _____

   _____

4. What might have contributed to this injury?

   _____

   _____

VOCABULARY

Match the word with its definition.

1. _____ Skin scraped away because of injury.
2. _____ Disease caused by an organism entering the body through an open wound that can cause lockjaw, seizures, abdominal rigidity, difficulty swallowing, breathing, and death.
3. _____ Insufficient intake of oxygen.
4. _____ Inadequate and progressively failing tissue perfusion that can result in cellular death.
5. _____ Irregular tear of the skin.
6. _____ Loss of water and electrolytes through heavy sweating, causing hypovolemia.
7. _____ Tearing away or crushing of body limbs.
8. _____ Frozen body parts that are white or yellow-white.
9. _____ A biological weapon that may occur in three forms: inhalational, cutaneous, and gastrointestinal.
10. _____ A biological weapon that can result in a severe febrile illness with hemoptysis as a classic sign.

1. Asphyxia
2. Tetanus
3. Abrasion
4. Laceration
5. Shock
6. Amputation
7. Heat exhaustion
8. Anthrax
9. Plague
10. Frostbite

PRINCIPLES FOR TREATING SHOCK

Indicate whether the statement is true or false and correct the false statement.

1. _____ Maintain an open airway.
2. _____ Give oxygen as ordered.
3. _____ Control external bleeding by indirect pressure.
4. _____ Apply cooling blanket to cool patient.
5. _____ If possible, keep the patient supine.
6. _____ Take hourly vital signs.
7. _____ Provide the patient with oral fluids.
8. _____ Monitor intravenous (IV) fluids as ordered.

SIGNS AND SYMPTOMS OF INCREASED INTRACRANIAL PRESSURE

Indicate whether the sign is an early sign or a late sign of increased intracranial pressure.

1. _____ Abnormal posturing

2. _____ Altered level of consciousness

3. _____ Amnesia

4. _____ Changes in respiratory pattern

5. _____ Changes in speech

6. _____ Decreased pulse rate

7. _____ Dilated nonreactive pupils

8. _____ Drowsiness

9. _____ Headache

10. _____ Nausea and vomiting

11. _____ Unresponsiveness

12. _____ Widening pulse pressure

1. Early sign

2. Late sign

ASSESSMENT OF MOTOR FUNCTION

Complete the table.

If the Patient is Unable to:	The Lesion is Above the Level of:
	C5 to C7
Extend and flex legs	
Flex foot, extend toes	
	S3 to S5

ENVIRONMENTAL HYPERTHERMIA

Indicate whether the sign is an early sign or a late sign of hyperthermia caused by exposure to a hot environment.

1. _____ Coma or seizures

2. _____ Diaphoresis

3. _____ Hot, dry, flushed skin

4. _____ Hypotension

5. _____ Pulse rate more than 100

6. _____ Dizziness

7. _____ Cool, clammy skin

8. _____ Altered mental status

9. _____ Core body temperature of 100.4° to 102.2°F
   (38° to 39°C)

10. _____ Core body temperature of 106°F (41°C) or more

1. Early sign

2. Late sign

PRINCIPLES FOR DISASTER OR BIOTERRORISM RESPONSE

Fill in the blank.

1. A disaster _____ existing personnel, facilities, and equipment.

2. Hospitals activate _____ plans in a disaster.

3. In a disaster, off-duty staff members are _____ to report to work, and noncritical patients are _____.

4. The emergency department serves as the _____ and _____ area.

5. Those treated first are the most _____ injured but who have the greatest chance for _____ recovery.

6. Disaster _____ are conducted on a regular basis.

7. You should be _____ with your _____ during a disaster.

8. Sources of disaster can include _____ agency events such as fires and explosions.

9. Floods, storms, fires, earthquakes, tornadoes, motor vehicle accidents, plane crashes, and acts of terrorism are _____ sources of disasters.

10. External disasters involve a _____ response of several agencies.

CRITICAL THINKING

Read the case study and answer the questions.

Mr. Harvey is a gardener. He is preparing the tractor to mow the lawn. He reaches down for a tool and is bitten by a snake. He immediately panics and runs to seek help from a neighbor.

1. What actions could the neighbor provide to assist with treatment of the patient?

_____

_____

_____

_____

2. What signs and symptoms would be exhibited with a poisonous (venomous) snakebite?

_____

_____

_____

_____

3. What treatment is appropriate for poisonous (venomous) snakebite?

_____

_____

_____

_____

4. What nursing diagnoses apply to Mr. Harvey?

_____

_____

_____

5. What nursing interventions are appropriate for Mr. Harvey? _____

_____

_____

_____

REVIEW QUESTIONS—CONTENT REVIEW

Choose the best answer unless directed otherwise.

1. For a patient who experiences anaphylactic shock after receiving a medication, which of the following symptoms would the nurse anticipate? **Select all that apply.**
   1. Chest pain
   2. Hot, dry skin
   3. Wheezing
   4. Fever
   5. Hypotension
   6. Stridor

2. The nurse is caring for a patient whose extremity may be fractured. Which of the following is the nurse's purpose in checking capillary refill of the extremity?
   1. To evaluate arterial blood flow in the extremity
   2. To evaluate venous blood flow in the extremity
   3. To measure oxygen saturation of the blood
   4. To identify peripheral edema

3. During data collection, which of the following findings would indicate to the nurse that severe blood loss has occurred?
   1. Normal, bounding pulse
   2. Slow, strong pulse
   3. Rapid, thready pulse
   4. Slow, bounding pulse

REVIEW QUESTIONS—TEST PREPARATION

Choose the best answer unless directed otherwise.

4. Which of the following monitoring is a priority for the nurse when caring for a patient with botulism exposure?
   1. Gag reflex
   2. Pupil response
   3. Corneal reflex
   4. Babinski response

5. The nurse anticipates that treatment for an unconscious patient who has ingested 50 tablets of alprazolam (Xanax), a noncaustic substance, could include which of the following?
   1. Administering an antiemetic
   2. Administering activated charcoal
   3. Administering an emetic
   4. Encouraging fluids

6. The nurse is caring for a patient who has hyperthermia. Which of the following indicates to the nurse that treatment has been effective?
   1. Skin is cool and moist to touch.
   2. Patient is alert and oriented.
   3. Core body temperature is less than 94°F (34.4°C).
   4. Core body temperature is greater than 101°F (38.3°C).

7. The health care provider orders haloperidol (Haldol) 3 mg intramuscularly for a patient who is experiencing a psychiatric crisis. Haloperidol 5 mg/mL is available. How many milliliters should the nurse give?
   1. 0.3 mL
   2. 0.5 mL
   3. 0.6 mL
   4. 1.3 mL

8. The nurse is collecting data on a patient with a large bleeding laceration. Which of the following vital sign data requires immediate action by the nurse?
   1. Thready pulse at 116
   2. Strong pulse at 84
   3. Regular pulse at 60
   4. Bounding pulse at 76

9. The nurse is admitting a trauma patient to the emergency department. Place in order of priority the areas for which data are collected as the nurse performs the primary survey. Use all options.
   1. Circulation
   2. Breathing
   3. Airway
   4. Disability
   5. Exposure

10. The nurse is caring for a patient who is bleeding from the radial artery. The nurse is applying direct pressure to the radial artery and has elevated the arm, but the wound continues to bleed. Which of the following actions should the nurse take immediately?
    1. Apply pressure to the carotid artery.
    2. Apply pressure to the brachial artery.
    3. Apply pressure to the femoral artery.
    4. Apply pressure to the temporal artery.

11. The nurse is caring for a patient after anthrax exposure who has a hemorrhagic, necrotic cutaneous lesion and is febrile. Which of the following items is important for the nurse to use while providing care to the patient? **Select all that apply.**
    1. Mask
    2. Gown
    3. Gloves
    4. Hair net
    5. Fit-tested N95 respirator
    6. Shoe covers

12. The nurse is caring for a patient with a narcotic overdose who is to receive naloxone (Narcan). Which observations of the patient would indicate to the nurse that the medication was effective? **Select all that apply.**
    1. No response to verbal stimuli
    2. Oriented to person and place
    3. Follows commands
    4. No response to painful stimuli
    5. Hand grasps equal and strong
    6. Pupils fixed

13. The nurse is caring for a patient who was submerged in fresh water and nearly drowned. The nurse would evaluate treatment as being effective if the patient exhibited which of the following? **Select all that apply.**
    1. Alertness
    2. Apnea
    3. Lethargy
    4. Tachypnea
    5. Respiratory rate of 16
    6. Regular respiratory pattern

14. A patient has a left leg laceration with bleeding that cannot be stopped. Mark the area where the nurse would apply pressure-point control to stop the bleeding.

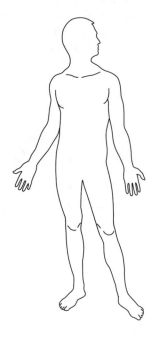

CHAPTER 14

Developmental Considerations and Chronic Illness in the Nursing Care of Adults

Name:
Date:
Course:
Instructor:

AUDIO CASE STUDY

Listen to the audio case study available on Davis Edge and then answer the following questions.

Julie and Older Adult Developmental Stages

1. What does Julie identify as the developmental task for Erikson's older adult stage?

   _____

   _____

2. How does Erikson define the task of integrity?

   _____

   _____

3. What task does Julie identify as Mr. Oscar needing to take on? Why?

   _____

   _____

   _____

4. What interventions does Julie plan to assist Mr. Oscar in working on this task?

   _____

   _____

   _____

VOCABULARY

Unscramble the word that fits the definition.

1. Short-term intermittent rest provided to caregivers—*serptei crea* _____

2. Perception that one's own actions will not affect an outcome—*wporelsesesns*

_____

3. Condition of long duration—*rhcnoic* _____

4. Life principles that pervade one's being—*sitrpiauilty* _____

5. State in which a person sees no alternatives or choices—*pohelesnsses* _____

6. A certain time frame during one's life containing tasks an individual needs to accomplish for high-level wellness—*evdlepoemnatl taseg* _____

CHRONIC ILLNESS AND THE OLDER ADULT

Find and correct the eight errors.

Older adults constitute one of the smallest age groups living with chronic illness. Older adult spouses or older family members rarely have to care for a chronically ill family member. Children of older adults who themselves are reaching their 40s are being expected to care for their parents. These older adult caregivers do not experience chronic illness themselves. For older adult spouses, it is usually the less ill spouse who provides care to the other spouse. The older adult family unit is at great risk for ineffective coping or further development of health problems. Nurses should collect data on ill members of the older adult family to ensure that their health needs are being met.

Older adults are not concerned about becoming dependent and a burden to others. They may become depressed and give up hope if they feel that they are a burden to others. Establishing long-term goals or self-care activities that allow them to participate or have small successes is an important nursing action that can decrease their self-esteem.

CRITICAL THINKING

Read the case study and answer the questions.

Mrs. Martin is hospitalized for an exacerbation of her multiple sclerosis. She tells the nurse she is tired of being ill and is not getting any better. She says, "When I am in the hospital, I cannot attend church, which is my only enjoyment." Later in the day, Mrs. Martin is tearful and withdrawn when the nurse makes rounds.

1. What further data collection should the nurse obtain to identify Mrs. Martin's patient-centered needs?

   _____

   _____

   _____

   _____

2. What possible nursing diagnoses would be appropriate for Mrs. Martin?

   _____

   _____

   _____

   _____

3. What patient-centered care interventions could the nurse use to assist Mrs. Martin in meeting her wish to attend church?

_____

_____

_____

_____

4. How would the nurse know that Mrs. Martin's goal has been met?

_____

_____

_____

_____

REVIEW QUESTIONS—CONTENT REVIEW

Choose the best answer unless directed otherwise.

1. The nurse is caring for a 72-year-old patient. When the nurse identifies the patient's developmental stage, which of the following of Erikson's developmental stages would the nurse expect the patient to be in?
   1. Generativity versus Self-Absorption
   2. Identity versus Role Confusion
   3. Intimacy versus Isolation
   4. Integrity versus Despair

2. Which of the following would the nurse anticipate finding for caregivers of patients who are chronically ill when respite care is not available?
   1. Personal time increases.
   2. Rest time increases.
   3. Financial costs increase.
   4. Stress levels increase.

3. The nurse is planning care for a patient with heart failure. Which of the following is a health promotion method the nurse can use that is helpful for this patient who is chronically ill?
   1. Making the choices for the patient.
   2. Setting the goals for the family.
   3. Setting the goals for the patient.
   4. Allowing the patient to make informed decisions.

4. The nurse is assigned to care for a group of patients with the following conditions. To plan patient-centered care, which of these does the nurse understand is an example of a chronic illness?
   1. Arthritis
   2. Bowel obstruction
   3. Cellulitis
   4. Peritonitis

5. Which of the following actions would a chronically ill patient need to perform in order for the nurse to evaluate him or her as fulfilling a primary task that those who are chronically ill need to perform?
   1. Being willing and able to carry out the medical regimen
   2. Reducing social activities to compensate for limitations
   3. Learning how to play the sick role
   4. Refusing to accept negative changes

6. The nurse is assigned to care for a group of patients. Which of these does the nurse understand is an example of a congenital chronic illness? **Select all that apply.**
   1. Head injury
   2. Malabsorption syndrome
   3. Emphysema
   4. Arthritis
   5. Cystic fibrosis
   6. Spina bifida

REVIEW QUESTIONS—TEST PREPARATION

Choose the best answer unless directed otherwise.

7. The nurse is developing a plan of care for a patient, age 68, focusing on preventive health care. While planning this care, the nurse understands that aging processes are most affected by which of the following factors?
   1. Stress management
   2. Financial issues
   3. Age at retirement
   4. Hobbies

8. A patient, age 64, is active and wants to learn health promotion interventions. Which of the following actions by the nurse supports the patient's desire for self-health promotion?
   1. Assign responsibilities for the patient's care to family members.
   2. Select a family physician for the patient.
   3. List health care activities for the patient to carry out.
   4. Ask the patient to choose desired health care activities.

9. The home health care nurse is caring for a patient with emphysema who seems depressed. Which of the following nursing interventions increases the patient's participation in self-care and assists with improving the patient's depression?
   1. Being a caregiver instead of a partner
   2. Assisting the patient
   3. Performing activities of daily living for the patient
   4. Doing everything for the patient

10. The nurse is caring for a patient who is recovering from a stroke. Which of the following nursing interventions during rehabilitation will increase the patient's self-esteem the most?
    1. Offering praise for small patient efforts
    2. Offering praise for major patient efforts
    3. Performing activities of daily living for the patient
    4. Assisting the patient at the first sign of difficulty with activities of daily living

11. Which of the following nursing actions might be most helpful for psychosocial intervention for the patient who is withdrawn, depressed, or tense because of isolation resulting from a chronic illness?
    1. Avoiding the use of humor
    2. Reading cartoons or jokes from magazines
    3. Maintaining a serious demeanor
    4. Limiting conversation to a minimum

12. In contributing to the plan of care for a patient who is chronically ill, which of the following is an appropriate nursing action designed to empower the patient?
    1. Provide educational information.
    2. Limit visiting hours for family members.
    3. Ask family members to provide care.
    4. Set goals for the patient and family.

13. The nurse is caring for a patient with Huntington disease. The family asks what the cause of the illness is. Which of the following responses is most appropriate by the nurse?
    1. "Huntington disease is a genetic disorder. Your family may want to consider genetic testing."
    2. "Huntington disease is a congenital disorder that developed in the womb."
    3. "Huntington disease is an acquired disorder caused by smoking."
    4. "Huntington disease is common among people over age 65, but the cause is unknown."

CHAPTER 15
Nursing Care of Older Adult Patients

Name:	_____
Date:	_____
Course:	_____
Instructor:	_____

AUDIO CASE STUDY

Listen to the audio case study available on Davis Edge and then answer the following questions.

Elise and the Older Adult

1. What changes occur in the urinary system with aging?

   _____

   _____

2. What effects do these changes have on urinary function?

   _____

   _____

   _____

   _____

3. What nursing interventions could be planned to provide patient-centered care when these urinary changes are experienced?

   _____

   _____

   _____

   _____

   _____

VOCABULARY

Fill in the blank with the word for the definition.

1. _____ Behaviors that are performed in the care and maintenance of self and surroundings

2. _____ Irregular heart rhythm

3. _____ Acute, reversible state of disorientation and confusion with difficulty focusing attention, inability to sleep, and hyperactivity due to an under- lying cause

4. _____ State of feeling or mind

5. _____ Accidental drawing of foreign substances into the airway

6. _____ Collection of excess fluid in body tissues

7. _____ Permanent progressive deterioration of mental function

8. _____ The act or process of coughing up materials from the air passageways leading to the lungs

9. _____ A condition of sluggish or difficult bowel action/evacuation

10. _____ The body's attempts to maintain a balance whenever a change occurs

11. _____ Abnormal accumulation of fibrosis connective tissue in skin, muscle, or joint capsule that prevents normal mobility

12. _____ An open sore or lesion of the skin that develops because of prolonged pressure against an area

13. _____ Excessive urination at night

14. _____ External variables that determine the occurrence and rate of structural and functional declines in the human body over time

15. _____ Factors that contribute to aging based on genetic and physiological theories of aging

16. _____ A condition in which there is a reduction in the mass of bone per unit volume

17. _____ None or minimal stimulation of senses that creates potential for maladaptive coping

18. _____ Highest level of patient activity considering the patient's condition

19. _____ A process to orient a person to names, dates, time, and other pertinent information through use of repeating messages

20. _____ Excessive stimulation of the senses that creates the potential for maladaptive coping

---

AGING CHANGES

Match the aging change with the effect of the change.

1. _____ Increased conduction time

2. _____ Decreased blood vessel elasticity

3. _____ Leg veins dilate, valves become less efficient

4. _____ Basal metabolic rate slows

5. _____ Decreased cardiac output

6. _____ Decreased insulin release

7. _____ Irregular heartbeats

8. _____ Altered adrenal hormone production

9. _____ Decreased gag reflex

10. _____ Decreased peristalsis

11. _____ Reduced liver enzymes

12. _____ Decreased saliva

1. Heart rate slows, unable to increase quickly

2. Less oxygen delivered to tissues

3. Increased blood pressure and cardiac workload

4. Poor heart oxygenation

5. Varicose veins, fluid accumulation in tissues

6. Possible weight gain

7. Decreased ability to respond to stress

8. Hyperglycemia

9. Appetite may be reduced

10. Dry mouth, altered taste

11. Increased aspiration risk

12. Frequency of urination

13. _____ Delayed gastric emptying

14. _____ Decreased bladder size and tone, changes from pear to funnel shaped

15. _____ Decreased kidney concentrating ability

16. _____ Decreased lung capacity

17. _____ Reduced kidney blood flow

18. _____ Decreased immune function

19. _____ Body content water loss

20. _____ Decreased sebaceous/sweat gland

21. _____ Reduced cell replacement

22. _____ Muscle responses slowed

23. _____ Decreased brain blood flow

24. _____ Less vaginal lubrication

25. _____ Decreased sensitivity

13. Reduced drug metabolism/detoxification

14. Reduced appetite, constipation

15. Painful intercourse

16. Nocturia

17. Greater infection and cancer risk

18. Decreased renal clearance of all medications

19. Slower healing process

20. Dryness of the skin

21. Decreased temperature regulation

22. Response time increased

23. Risk of injury, burns

24. Dyspnea with activity

25. Short-term memory loss

COMMUNICATING WITH PEOPLE WHO HAVE HEARING IMPAIRMENTS

Indicate whether the statement is true or false and correct false statements.

1. _____ Ensure that hearing aids are turned on and have working batteries.

2. _____ The speaker should turn to the side so the speaker's profile is visible to the patient.

3. _____ Speak toward the patient's impaired side of hearing.

4. _____ Speak in a clear, soft to moderate volume and low-pitched tone.

5. _____ Do not shout because doing so distorts sounds.

6. _____ High-frequency tones and consonant sounds are lost last (e.g., *s, z, sh, ch, d, g*).

7. _____ Eliminate background noise because it distorts sounds.

MEDICATIONS

Find the six errors and correct them.

Older patients are less susceptible to drug-induced illness and adverse medication side effects for various reasons. They take few medicines for the one chronic illness that they have. Different medications interact and produce side effects that can be dangerous. Over-the-counter medicines that older patients take as well as the self-prescribed extracts, elixirs, herbal teas, cultural healing substances, and other home remedies commonly used by individuals of their age cohort do not influence other medications.

If an older patient crushes a large enteric-coated pill so that it can be taken in food for easy swallowing it enhances the enteric protection and can inadvertently cause damage to the stomach and intestinal system. Some patients unintentionally skip prescribed doses in an effort to save money. When prescribed doses are not being taken as expected, problems do not clear up as quickly, and new problems may result. The nurse should educate the older patient and the patient's family. Patients need to know what each prescribed pill is for, when it is prescribed to be taken, and how it should be taken.

CRITICAL THINKING

Read the following case study and answer the questions. This is a values clarification exercise.

While making 2200 rounds in the long-term care facility, the nurse looks into Mr. Braun's room to find him and a female resident from down the hall sleeping soundly together in Mr. Braun's bed. Mr. Braun and the female resident are both 76 years of age. Mr. Shaw, who is Mr. Braun's roommate, is sound asleep alone in his own bed.

1. What are your initial feelings about this situation?

   _____

   _____

   _____

   _____

2. What influences your feelings? _____

   _____

   _____

   _____

3. What is the first thing that you would do after this discovery? _____

   _____

   _____

4. What issues should you consider before making a decision?

   _____

   _____

   _____

5. How will you interact with these patients in the future?

   _____

   _____

   _____

REVIEW QUESTIONS—CONTENT REVIEW

Choose the best answer unless directed otherwise.

1. Which of the following does the nurse recognize as an aging change in the cardiovascular system?
   1. Increased cardiac output
   2. Increased peripheral vascular resistance
   3. Increased resting heart rate
   4. Increased cardiac reserve

2. The nurse understands that which of the following factors is most often the cause of sexual dysfunction for older people?
   1. Physical factors
   2. Psychological factors
   3. Social factors
   4. Environmental factors

3. Which of the following actions should the older adult take to prevent osteoporosis?
   1. Decrease dietary intake of calcium.
   2. Commit to regular exercise.
   3. Increase dietary intake of salt.
   4. Increase dietary protein intake.

REVIEW QUESTIONS—TEST PREPARATION

Choose the best answer unless directed otherwise.

4. As the nurse collects data on an 84-year-old patient, which of the following is an expected finding within the patient's mouth caused by advancing age?
   1. Loss of teeth
   2. Hardness of the gums
   3. Increased production of saliva
   4. Decreased taste sensitivity for salt

5. Which of the following does the nurse understand is the rationale for assisting a 70-year-old patient to sit on the bedside before standing?
   1. To provide a heightened awareness of body position
   2. To accommodate a less efficient circulatory system
   3. To strengthen legs
   4. To reduce anxiety about getting up

6. The nurse provides care to an 80-year-old patient with an intravenous infusion. The nurse understands that it is essential for older patients who are receiving intravenous fluids to be monitored closely to prevent which of the following?
   1. Circulatory overload
   2. Dislodging of the intravenous line
   3. Venous distention
   4. Increased urinary output

7. The nurse is talking with a patient who is hard of hearing and having difficulty with high-pitched tones. Which of the following actions should the nurse take when speaking with the patient?
   1. Speak slowly with emphasis on important words.
   2. Double the voice volume.
   3. Whisper responses in proximity to the patient's ear.
   4. Use a modulated voice and talk normally in either ear.

8. A nurse is working in a long-term care facility. Which of the following nursing behaviors demonstrates the nurse's respect for the older patient's sexuality?
   1. Providing private time by ensuring that the patient is undisturbed for an hour
   2. Entering a patient's room without knocking when a visitor is present
   3. Entering the room to prepare medications while a patient and visitor are embracing
   4. Changing the subject when a patient expresses personal feelings toward a friend

9. The nurse recognizes that which of the following older patients would be at highest risk for using inappropriate prescription medication?
   1. A 60-year-old college professor recently diagnosed with diabetes admitted with cellulitis
   2. A 72-year-old with a ninth-grade education who suffered double below-the-knee amputations in the Korean War admitted with a decubitus ulcer
   3. A 76-year-old retired lawyer with a history of hypertension and chronic kidney failure admitted for dehydration
   4. An 81-year-old retired teacher with a history of colorectal cancer admitted for a colonoscopy

10. The nurse explains gentle bathing techniques to the nursing assistant. The nurse would evaluate the nursing assistant as understanding the teaching if the assistant stated which of these? **Select all that apply**.
    1. "The towel bath provides gentle bathing."
    2. "A glove bath can be used for gentle bathing."
    3. "Gentle forms of bathing are drying to the skin."
    4. "Hot water and soap are used for gentle bathing."
    5. "Gentle bathing protects the skin of the older adult."

CHAPTER 16
Patient Care Settings

Name:	_____
Date:	_____
Course:	_____
Instructor:	_____

AUDIO CASE STUDY

Listen to the audio case study available on Davis Edge and then answer the following questions.

Shawn and Home Health Care

1. When the nurse is preparing for home visits, what should be considered in developing an efficient schedule to see the patients?

   _____

   _____

   _____

   _____

2. When visiting a patient who is taking warfarin (Coumadin), what diet information should the nurse be prepared to teach and answer patient questions related to the influence of diet on warfarin (Coumadin) and INR/PT levels?

   _____

   _____

3. How does the Internet help the nurse plan for a safe home visit?

   _____

   _____

   _____

   _____

VOCABULARY

Match the term to the correct definition.

1. _____ Autonomous
2. _____ Triage
3. _____ Chemical restraint
4. _____ Collaborative care
5. _____ Community resources
6. _____ Homebound
7. _____ Private-duty
8. _____ Respite care
9. _____ Skilled nursing
10. _____ Physical restraint
11. _____ Telenursing
12. _____ OASIS
13. _____ Acute Care for Elders units
14. _____ Long-term care services
15. _____ Elopement

1. Care that can only be delivered by a licensed professional nurse
2. Occurs when a patient is unable to leave his or her home to obtain necessary health care services
3. To work together to achieve a goal
4. Assignment of degree of urgency to decide the order of treatment of patients
5. Use of medication to restrict the freedom or movement of a person
6. To work independently
7. Available to a home health care patient to improve his or her quality of care; usually coordinated by a social worker
8. Scheduled care to assist the patient with personal and homemaking needs
9. Any manual method or device, material, or equipment attached to or near the body that can't easily be removed
10. Provides family members and caregivers time to take care of themselves
11. Health and nonhealth care services for those who are disabled or frail
12. Leaving a facility unsupervised when unable to protect oneself
13. Design meets unique needs of hospitalized older adults to prevent functional decline
14. Information technology and telecommunication to provide nursing care
15. Outcome and Assessment Information Set

HOME HEALTH CARE SERVICES

Match the home health care team member's role to the appropriate definition.

1. _____ Social worker
2. _____ Physical therapist
3. _____ Occupational therapist
4. _____ Registered nurse
5. _____ Home health care aide
6. _____ Licensed practical nurse/licensed vocational nurse (LPN/LVN)
7. _____ Speech therapist
8. _____ Health care provider

1. Assists the patient with activities of daily living (ADLs)
2. Develops the plan of care and manages the care of the patient during home health care services
3. Assists the patient with access to community resources
4. Assists the patient with developing independence with ADLs
5. Assists the patient with strength and gait training
6. Assists the patient with language, speech, or swallowing
7. Team leader
8. Makes home visits and performs skilled nursing care

PATIENT CARE SETTING LPN/LVN DUTIES

Match the duty/action of an LPN/LVN to the patient care setting for the nursing duty/action.

1. _____ Greet, triage, and register patients
2. _____ Respond to emergencies as health care team member
3. _____ Companionship and respite care
4. _____ Teach residents and families
5. _____ Assist with renewal of prescriptions
6. _____ Assist with end-of-life care and medication review
7. _____ Provide precertification and coordination for inmates admitted to and discharged from acute care facilities
8. _____ Fill weekly medication dispensers
9. _____ Evaluate environment for patient's safety
10. _____ Display sensitivity to cultural and socioeconomic differences among populace related to health and behaviors
11. _____ Monitor residents to prevent and detect pressure injury
12. _____ Video/audio conference to collect patient data
13. _____ Plan for personal safety
14. _____ Obtain prior authorization of medications
15. _____ Use patient's bathroom to wash hands

1. Correctional facility
2. Home health care agency
3. Long-term care facility
4. Medical office
5. Private-duty
6. Telenursing

CRITICAL THINKING

Read the following case study and answer the questions.

Mrs. Thompson was just discharged from the hospital after an exacerbation of her respiratory disease. Her health history includes chronic obstructive pulmonary disease, type 2 diabetes, and coronary artery disease. She is receiving oxygen (O_2) therapy at 2 L/minute via nasal cannula. She has a skin tear on her right lower extremity requiring dressing changes every other day for 4 weeks. The health care provider prescribed a beta blocker for heart rate control.

Mrs. Thompson lives alone and verbalized to the registered nurse on admission that it is difficult for her to prepare meals and "get around the house." She has one married daughter who lives locally and works full-time.

1. How often will Mrs. Thompson require skilled nursing services? _____
_____
_____

2. What services will the home health nurse be performing?
_____
_____
_____
_____

3. What are safety considerations for Mrs. Thompson?
_____
_____
_____
_____

4. Would Mrs. Thompson benefit from any other home health care services?
_____
_____
_____
_____

REVIEW QUESTIONS—CONTENT REVIEW

Choose the best answer unless directed otherwise.

1. The nurse is orienting to the home health care agency and learns the roles of team members for collaborative care. Which of these members of the home health care team would the nurse anticipate interacting with to provide collaborative care? **Select all that apply.**
   1. Registered nurse
   2. Health care provider
   3. Social worker
   4. Home health aide
   5. Lawyer
   6. Patient

2. When providing care to a patient in the patient's home, the nurse understands that which of the following persons is in control of the home health care environment?
   1. Family
   2. Health care provider
   3. Nurse
   4. Patient

REVIEW QUESTIONS—TEST PREPARATION

Choose the best answer unless directed otherwise.

3. The home health nurse is making a first-time visit to a patient at home. Which of the following techniques could the nurse use to develop trust with the patient?
   1. Review patient's history to plan patient needs before visit.
   2. Call the night before the visit to set a time for the visit.
   3. Acknowledge the patient's fears that are expressed.
   4. Discuss treatment plans with the patient only.

4. The home health nurse collects safety data on an initial visit to the home of a patient who has returned from the hospital and has an infected abdominal wound requiring dressing changes. Which of the following interventions should the nurse include in the plan of care to promote safety in the home? **Select all that apply.**
   1. Explain to the patient never to get out of bed without assistance.
   2. Instruct a family member to be available at all times to assist with ambulation.
   3. Clean the patient's home each visit to maintain asepsis.
   4. Instruct the family to remove all scatter rugs.
   5. Ask family to install handrails in the hallway for ambulation.
   6. Clear walkways of all clutter.

5. The home health nurse arrives at a patient's home. Which of the following interventions performed by the nurse demonstrate understanding of the importance of following infection control principles in the home?
   1. Setting the nurse's home health care bag on the floor
   2. Cleaning supplies after each home health care visit
   3. Washing hands in the patient's kitchen sink
   4. Using dressing supplies sitting open on a table

6. The nurse is to give a patient 8 mg of intramuscular morphine for pain. The nurse has available 10 mg of morphine/mL. How many mL will the nurse give? _____ mL

7. The home health nurse is making a home visit to a 68-year-old patient and is reinforcing medication teaching that was done in the hospital setting. The nurse understands that the teaching will be more effective with which of the following techniques? **Select all that apply.**
   1. Provide a long teaching session.
   2. Include a support person.
   3. Make instructions simple.
   4. Provide demonstration.
   5. Repeat instructions often.

8. The home health nurse is visiting a patient to check blood glucose and administer insulin. As the nurse obtains the insulin from the refrigerator where the patient stores it, the nurse observes that dirty dishes are stacked in the kitchen sink and that there is only a moldy open can of soup, a sandwich, and cat food in the refrigerator. Which of the following actions should the nurse take regarding the visit findings?
   1. Inform the registered nurse of the moldy and sparse food.
   2. Tell the patient to wash the dishes.
   3. Notify the registered nurse that the patient is eating cat food.
   4. Wash the dirty dishes.

9. Which of the following could the home health nurse do to prepare for a home health care visit and ensure that it is a safe and effective visit? **Select all that apply.**
   1. Keep cell phone battery charged.
   2. Provide an exact time for arrival.
   3. Obtain driving directions to the patient's home.
   4. Park in the patient's driveway.
   5. Keep gas tank filled.
   6. Carry a whistle.

10. The registered nurse is visiting an 89-year-old woman at home to assess the need for skilled nursing care after a fall resulting in a broken collarbone. Which of the following should be included in the nurse's initial visit? **Select all that apply.**
    1. Identify fall risks in the home environment.
    2. Observe the patient performing activities of daily living.
    3. Collect baseline vital signs.
    4. Obtain a urine sample for culture and sensitivity.
    5. Review patient medications and their schedule.

11. A nurse has begun working for a local home health care agency and is concerned about the transition to home health care nursing after working in the hospital for 10 years. What recommendations by a supervisor would ease this transition for the nurse? **Select all that apply.**
    1. Explain that home health care nursing is the same as hospital nursing.
    2. Explain that being prepared and keeping paperwork organized is essential.
    3. Discuss feelings about the transition and ask questions.
    4. Let the nurse know it is not possible to completely adjust to home health care nursing because of variability across homes.
    5. Spend time the day before a visit to review patient health information to help gain confidence in the home.

12. A patient has just been discharged from the hospital after open heart surgery. The patient's spouse is the primary caregiver and confides that handling all of the finances, managing the patient's complex medication regime, assisting with activities of daily living, and generally managing the household is a concern. Which of the following would be an appropriate nursing diagnosis for the patient's spouse?
    1. *Ineffective Coping*
    2. *Powerlessness*
    3. *Ineffective Health Maintenance*
    4. *Risk for Caregiver Role Strain*

13. A licensed practical nurse is to interview for a position in a medical office and is reviewing the job description. Which of these tasks for this role would be included in the job description? **Select all that apply.**
    1. Develop the plan of care.
    2. Enter data into the electronic medical record.
    3. Escort patients to examination rooms.
    4. Provide patient care (such as wound care, dressings).
    5. Monitor patients after medications or treatments.
    6. Document understanding of teaching.

14. A nurse orients to a new position in a correctional facility by learning which of the following? **Select all that apply.**
    1. Institutional quality standards, procedures, and protocols
    2. Cultural and socioeconomic differences for health care among the populace
    3. Postcertification for inmate admission to acute care facilities
    4. Provision of empathy to inmates during treatments
    5. Role in responding to health care emergencies
    6. Cardiopulmonary resuscitation

15. The nurse is providing information to a patient's caregiver on long-term care services. Which of these settings would the nurse include as providing long-term care services? **Select all that apply.**
    1. Adult day-care service center
    2. Assisted living facility
    3. Patient's home
    4. Hospital
    5. Memory care facility
    6. Residential care community

16. What action can the nurse take related to the environment of a patient with dementia to increase the patient's quality of life?
    1. Decrease bright lighting
    2. Reduce noise
    3. Keep window blinds closed
    4. Provide background noise

17. The nurse is contributing to the plan of care for a patient who is being admitted to an assisted living facility. What interventions can the nurse include to promote patient safety in long-term care? **Select all that apply.**
    1. Stretching exercises
    2. Well-lit environment
    3. Provide adequate vitamin D intake
    4. A review of medications for side effects
    5. Limit calcium intake

CHAPTER 17
Nursing Care of Patients at the End of Life

Name:	
Date:	
Course:	
Instructor:	

AUDIO CASE STUDY

Listen to the audio case study available on Davis Edge and then answer the following questions.

Mr. Sellers at the End of His Life

1. What is a durable medical power of attorney? A living will?

   _____
   _____
   _____
   _____
   _____

2. When do these documents take effect?

   _____
   _____

3. What signs did Mr. Sellers exhibit that indicated he was approaching the end of life?

   _____
   _____

VOCABULARY

Fill in the blank.

1. One part of an advance directive includes a document instructing caregivers in patients' medical preferences at end of life, called a _____.

2. A _____ document specifies who can make decisions for a patient when the patient can no longer make decisions.

3. Patients qualify for _____ care when their prognosis is 6 months or less.

4. Care of the body after death is called _____ care.

5. The nurse who communicates patients' and families' wishes to the health care team is acting as a patient

_____.

TRUE OR FALSE?

Indicate whether the statement is true or false and correct false statements.

1. _____ Older adult patients usually gain weight while undergoing treatment in a hospital.

2. _____ Only a few health insurance companies provide a hospice benefit.

3. _____ Insomnia, headaches, and fatigue can be a sign of grief in nurses.

4. _____ Dehydration in dying patients causes endorphins to be released that will enhance comfort.

5. _____ Patients who live longer than 6 months while on hospice will be discharged from the hospice program.

6. _____ Terminal illness is experienced by the whole family.

7. _____ To improve the chance of success for patients receiving cardiopulmonary resuscitation (CPR) at the time of cardiac arrest, CPR must be started within 8 minutes.

8. _____ One benefit of withholding artificial fluids in patients who are actively dying is fewer pharyngeal and lung secretions.

9. _____ Eighty percent of communication with terminal patients and their families is nonverbal.

10. _____ Confusion and agitation are two common indicators that older adult patients are approaching the end of life.

CRITICAL THINKING

Read the following case study and answer the questions.

Your patient, Mrs. Brown, is actively dying from end-stage lung cancer. List at least two nursing interventions that may be helpful to treat each symptom she is experiencing:

1. Dyspnea _____

_____

_____

2. Bowel and bladder incontinence _____

_____

_____

3. Copious oral secretions _____

_____

_____

4. Body temperature changes _____

_____

_____

5. Restlessness _____

_____

_____

REVIEW QUESTIONS—CONTENT REVIEW

Choose the best answer unless directed otherwise.

1. Research on patients with dementia who received tube feedings revealed which of the following risks?
   1. The risk of pain was increased.
   2. The risk of aspiration was increased.
   3. The risk of excess weight gain increased.
   4. The risk of pressure ulcers increased.

2. What question can be most effective in finding out the patient's understanding of the severity of the illness the patient is experiencing?
   1. "How do you feel about your illness?"
   2. "How is your family coping with your illness?"
   3. "What has the doctor told you about your illness?"
   4. "What would you like to do about your illness?"

3. A dying patient's family members are upset and crying. Which action by the nurse will best help the family?
   1. Sustain eye contact and encourage them to talk about their concerns.
   2. Ask them to speak quietly so as not to disturb the other patients.
   3. Tell them that, for the sake of their loved one, they need to compose themselves.
   4. Move them to another room away from the patient.

REVIEW QUESTIONS—TEST PREPARATION

Choose the best answer unless directed otherwise.

4. A family member asks why a dying patient is receiving morphine when the patient doesn't appear to be in any pain. Which response by the nurse is best?
   1. "Morphine helps make patients less aware of their surroundings."
   2. "Morphine helps patients breathe more comfortably."
   3. "Morphine helps keep body temperature under control."
   4. "Morphine helps patients sleep."

5. A patient has just been pronounced dead. What is the first action the nurse should take?
   1. Contact the nursing supervisor.
   2. Remove the patient's tubes and create a clean, peaceful impression for the family.
   3. Make sure the patient gets to the funeral home within 12 hours for embalming.
   4. Move the patient out of the hospital room to the morgue.

6. A dying patient appears confused and keeps saying he sees his wife who died 10 years earlier. The family appears upset by this. What teaching should the nurse provide?
   1. Teach them to redirect the patient and gently remind him that his wife died long ago.
   2. Explain that this happens because of the medications that the patient is receiving.
   3. Explain that this is a common occurrence and encourage them to allow him to talk about his experience.
   4. Explain that this can occur when the brain is deprived of oxygen and then get an order for oxygen if the patient does not already have it.

7. An older patient with chronic disease is very weak and chokes when attempting to eat. The patient's daughter is upset and wants a feeding tube inserted. The physician has told her that the patient is dying and that a tube will not prolong life. The daughter is now crying in the hallway. Which response by the nurse is best?
   1. Reiterate what the doctor said about the patient not living any longer with a tube.
   2. Tell the daughter that a tube is uncomfortable for the patient.
   3. Tell the daughter the staff will feed the patient more slowly to prevent choking.
   4. Acknowledge how hard this is for her, as she has taken such good care of feeding the patient throughout the illness.

8. A patient being discharged from the hospital has decided she does not want to be resuscitated should she experience a cardiopulmonary arrest at home. Which of the following documents should the nurse assist the patient to complete?
   1. Living will
   2. Advance medical directive
   3. Durable power of attorney
   4. Physician orders for life-sustaining treatment

9. The family members of a patient who is terminally ill ask a nurse if they may bathe their loved one after death, in keeping with their cultural traditions. Which response is best?
   1. "You should concentrate on the time you have left together."
   2. "Your cultural traditions are important and will be supported by our staff."
   3. "Our staff will make sure the patient is clean and bathed."
   4. "That won't be necessary, because the funeral home takes care of bathing the patient."

10. The family members of a patient with terminal cancer have agreed to stop aggressive treatment and begin comfort measures only. Which of the following statements would the nurse include in a discussion of specific decisions? **Select all that apply.**
    1. "Withholding artificial hydration can make breathing more comfortable."
    2. "Pain may be reduced if artificial hydration is stopped because tumor swelling is decreased."
    3. "If the intravenous fluids are stopped, the patient's body will stop making endorphins."
    4. "Research indicates that tube feeding in people dying of cancer is not beneficial."
    5. "Patients who are not fed often say they are hungry as they are dying."

CHAPTER 18
Immune System Function, Assessment, and Therapeutic Measures

Name: _____

Date: _____

Course: _____

Instructor: _____

AUDIO CASE STUDY

Listen to the audio case study available on Davis Edge and then answer the following questions.

Scott and Anaphylaxis

1. How might those with food allergies be exposed to the food allergen?

_____

_____

_____

2. What should someone with a food allergy always have as a precaution?

_____

_____

3. What symptoms of an allergic reaction did Scott experience?

_____

_____

4. What actions did Scott and his brother take that put Scott's health in jeopardy?

_____

_____

_____

_____

STRUCTURES OF THE IMMUNE SYSTEM

Label the following structures.

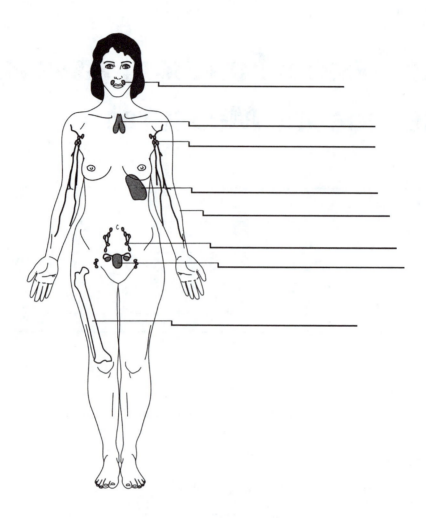

IMMUNE SYSTEM CELLS

Match each cell of the immune system with the correct description.

1. _____ Memory cells
2. _____ Helper T cells
3. _____ Cytotoxic T cells
4. _____ Plasma cells
5. _____ Suppressor T cells
6. _____ Macrophages
7. _____ B cells

1. Phagocytize pathogens labeled with antibodies
2. Produce antibodies
3. Limit the immune response once the pathogen has been destroyed
4. Initiate a rapid immune response if the pathogen reenters the body
5. Destroy cells directly by lysing their membranes
6. May become plasma cells or memory cells
7. Participate in antigen recognition and activate B cells

ANTIBODIES

Name the proper class of antibodies for each of these functions.

1. Found in mucous membrane secretions _____

2. Provides long-term immunity _____

3. Forms the receptors on B cells _____

4. Important in allergic reactions _____

5. Crosses the placenta to fetal circulation _____

6. Found in breast milk _____

7. The first antibody produced in an infection _____

VOCABULARY

Fill in the blank.

1. _____ are chemical markers that identify cells or molecules.

2. _____ is the ability to destroy pathogens or other foreign material and to prevent further cases of certain infectious diseases.

3. _____, _____, and _____ are the three types of lymphocytes.

4. _____ mature in the thymus gland.

5. _____ are also called antibodies.

6. _____ immunity is the type of immunity that involves only T cells.

7. _____ immunity is the type of immunity in which a person has recovered from a disease and now has antibodies and memory cells specific for that pathogen.

8. The immunoglobulin _____ provides long-term immunity following recovery from an illness.

9. Lymph node enlargement with tenderness is usually indicative of _____ and infection.

10. The _____ of a white blood cell differential are increased in bacterial infections.

IMMUNE SYSTEM

Match the word with the definition.

1. _____ Allergy shots

2. _____ Confirmation test for HIV-1 if antigen/antibody combination immunoassay is positive but antibody differentiation immunoassay is nonreactive or inconclusive.

3. _____ Important in allergic reactions and attaches to mast cells

4. _____ Swelling around the eyes

5. _____ A test done to confirm a diagnosis, determine a prognosis, or evaluate effectiveness of treatment

6. _____ Found in secretions of all mucous membranes

7. _____ Itching

1. Periorbital edema

2. Biopsy

3. Pruritus

4. Nucleic acid test

5. IgE

6. C-reactive protein

7. Immunotherapy

8. _____ An abnormal protein found in plasma during an acute inflammatory process

9. _____ Detects both HIV-1 and HIV-2 antibodies and HIV-1 p24 antigen

10. _____ Differentiates between HIV-1 and HIV-2 antibodies

8. IgA

9. Antibody differentiation immunoassay

10. Antigen/antibody combination immunoassay

DATA COLLECTION—HISTORY

Find and correct the eight errors in the following two paragraphs.

Demographic Data

The patient's age, gender, race, and ethnic background is important data. Systemic lupus erythematosus affects men ten times more frequently than women. The patient's place of birth gives insight into ethnic ties. Where the patient has lived and does live may shed light on the current illness. The patient's occupation, such as that of a coal miner, may contribute to gastrointestinal symptoms.

History

Food, medication, and environmental allergies should include those that the patient experiences and those present in the family history. With a family history, a previous exposure to a substance is required before a severe reaction occurs. Conditions such as allergic rhinitis, systemic lupus erythematosus, ankylosing spondylitis, and asthma are thought to be either familial or have a congenital predisposition.

If the patient's thymus gland has been removed (thymectomy), B-cell production may be altered. Corticosteroids and immunosuppressants enhance the immune response. The patient's lifestyle may place the patient at low risk for contracting the human immunodeficiency virus.

CRITICAL THINKING

Read the following case study and answer the questions.

David Case, age 29, is visiting his health care provider because he has been extremely fatigued for several months and now has swollen lymph nodes in his neck. On palpation, the area feels enlarged, nontender, hard, and fixed.

1. What categories of data collection should the nurse obtain? _____
   _____
   _____
   _____

2. What might the palpation findings indicate?_____
   _____
   _____
   _____

3. What categories of data collection would be important to explore in detail? _____
   _____
   _____
   _____

REVIEW QUESTIONS—CONTENT REVIEW

Choose the best answer unless directed otherwise.

1. A baby is born temporarily immune to the diseases to which the mother is immune. The nurse would explain this to the mother as being which of the following types of immunity?
   1. Naturally acquired passive immunity
   2. Artificially acquired passive immunity
   3. Naturally acquired active immunity
   4. Artificially acquired active immunity

2. Immunity to a disease after recovery is possible because the first exposure to the pathogen has stimulated the formation of which of the following?
   1. Antigens
   2. Memory cells
   3. Complement
   4. Natural killer cells

3. Which of the following immunoglobulins is first produced during an acute infection?
   1. IgD
   2. IgE
   3. IgG
   4. IgM

4. Which of the following is the function of macrophages and neutrophils?
   1. Phagocytosis
   2. Antibody production
   3. Complement fixation
   4. Suppression of autoimmunity

5. The activation of B cells in humoral immunity is assisted by which of the following?
   1. Cytotoxic T cells
   2. Helper T cells
   3. Suppressor T cells
   4. Neutrophils

6. *Autoimmunity* is defined as a phenomenon involving which of the following?
   1. Production of endotoxins that destroy B lymphocytes
   2. Inability to differentiate self from nonself
   3. Overproduction of reagin antibody
   4. Depression of the immune response

REVIEW QUESTIONS—TEST PREPARATION

Choose the best answer unless directed otherwise.

7. Which of the following is used to determine the presence of inflammation? **Select all that apply.**
   1. IgM assay
   2. CD4+ count
   3. Western blot
   4. C-reactive protein
   5. Erythrocyte sedimentation rate

8. A mother brings her children into the clinic, and the children are diagnosed with chickenpox. The mother had chickenpox as a child. Which of the following statements should the nurse include in the patient teaching?
   1. "Because you have an active natural immunity to chickenpox, you can take care of the children at home."
   2. "You will need to wear a mask while caring for the children to prevent contamination."
   3. "You will need to get a booster chickenpox vaccination to ensure that you don't get reinfected."
   4. "Because you've had chickenpox before and your children are now ill, you should monitor yourself for signs or symptoms of shingles for the next 2 weeks."

9. The nurse is teaching a patient about immune function. Which of the following would the nurse correctly include as stimulating antibody production? Select all that apply.
   1. Cold virus
   2. Plant pollen
   3. Transplanted organ
   4. Bacterial toxins
   5. Measles vaccine

10. The nurse is caring for a patient undergoing a biopsy. Which action is appropriate for the nurse to take?
    1. Ask whether the patient has an iodine allergy.
    2. Ensure that informed consent is obtained before the procedure.
    3. Ask the patient about environmental allergies and the type of reaction that occurs.
    4. Check eosinophil level on the laboratory report.

11. While working with patients in an autoimmune disease clinic, the nurse recognizes that which of the following individuals is most likely to develop systemic lupus erythematosus?
    1. A 38-year-old African American male who works in the construction industry
    2. A 55-year-old Caucasian female who works as a medical secretary
    3. A 19-year-old Asian female who is attending college
    4. A 34-year-old Native American male who works as a lawyer

CHAPTER 19
Nursing Care of Patients With Immune Disorders

Name:	_____
Date:	_____
Course:	_____
Instructor:	_____

AUDIO CASE STUDY

Listen to the audio case study available on Davis Edge and then answer the following questions.

Ayla and Systemic Lupus Erythematosus

1. What are three types of lupus in adults?

   _____

   _____

2. Who is more prone to developing systemic lupus erythematosus (SLE)?

   _____

   _____

3. What precautions will Ayla need to take to help control the disease and its symptoms?

   _____

   _____

   _____

   _____

VOCABULARY

Match the term with its definition.

1. _____ An anaphylactic-type reaction
2. _____ The type of antibodies that attach to mast cells
3. _____ Results from antigen–antibody reaction
4. _____ Very dry, pruritic, edematous skin
5. _____ Sudden, severe reaction characterized by smooth muscle spasms and capillary permeability changes
6. _____ Urticaria
7. _____ A form of lupus that affects only the skin
8. _____ Types of drugs used to prevent transplant rejection
9. _____ Painless subcutaneous and dermal erythemic eruptions with diffuse edema
10. _____ Requires lifelong vitamin B$_{12}$
11. _____ Red blood cell fragments seen with microscope
12. _____ Absence or deficiency of one or more immunoglobulin (Ig)G, IgM, IgA, IgD, and IgE from defective B-cell function
13. _____ Antimalarial and immunosuppressant drugs may be used in treatment
14. _____ Causes may include heat, cold, pressure, and stress
15. _____ Patient education includes a diet low in iodine and high in bulk, protein, and carbohydrates
16. _____ Patient education includes frequent movement and the use of a hard mattress and no or thin pillow when sleeping

1. Urticaria
2. Angioedema
3. Anaphylaxis
4. Pernicious anemia
5. Hashimoto's thyroiditis
6. Idiopathic autoimmune hemolytic anemia
7. Hypogammaglobulinemia
8. Allergic rhinitis
9. Hives
10. Type I hypersensitivity reaction
11. IgE
12. Ankylosing spondylitis
13. Atopic dermatitis
14. Immunosuppressive
15. Systemic lupus erythematosus
16. Discoid lupus erythematosus

IMMUNE DISORDERS

Fill in the blank.

1. Hypersensitivity reactions are classified as _____,
   _____, _____, and _____.

2. When allergic rhinitis occurs seasonally, it is called _____.

3. Complications of allergic rhinitis are _____, _____,
   _____, and _____.

4. _____ is a complication of atopic dermatitis.

5. The first drug of choice for anaphylaxis is _____.

6. Urticaria is commonly called _____.

7. Angioedema differs from urticaria in that angioedema is _____ and lasts
   _____.

8. The _____ is used to diagnose a hemolytic transfusion reaction.

9. _____ and _____ are
   two complications that can occur with a hemolytic transfusion reaction.

10. Today, serum sickness tends to occur when _____ and
    _____ are administered to patients.

11. _____ and _____ are two food additives that can trigger
    an anaphylactic reaction.

12. _____ is the most common cause of contact dermatitis.

13. Patients with pernicious anemia are unable to absorb _____.

14. _____ is a process whereby abnormal red blood cells are removed and replaced
    with normal red blood cells.

15. Ankylosing spondylitis is a chronic progressive inflammatory disease of the
    _____, _____, and large _____
    joints.

IMMUNE WORD SEARCH

Figure out what words the clues represent. Then find the words in the grid. Words can go horizontally, vertically, and diagonally in all eight directions.

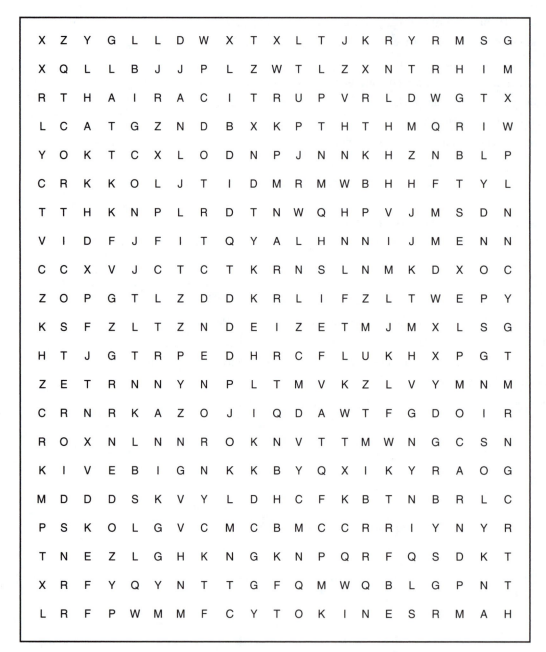

```
X  Z  Y  G  L  L  D  W  X  T  X  L  T  J  K  R  Y  R  M  S  G
X  Q  L  L  B  J  J  P  L  Z  W  T  L  Z  X  N  T  R  H  I  M
R  T  H  A  I  R  A  C  I  T  R  U  P  V  R  L  D  W  G  T  X
L  C  A  T  G  Z  N  D  B  X  K  P  T  H  T  H  M  Q  R  I  W
Y  O  K  T  C  X  L  O  D  N  P  J  N  N  K  H  Z  N  B  L  P
C  R  K  K  O  L  J  T  I  D  M  R  M  W  B  H  H  F  T  Y  L
T  T  H  K  N  P  L  R  D  T  N  W  Q  H  P  V  J  M  S  D  N
V  I  D  F  J  F  I  T  Q  Y  A  L  H  N  N  I  J  M  E  N  N
C  C  X  V  J  C  T  C  T  K  R  N  S  L  N  M  K  D  X  O  C
Z  O  P  G  T  L  Z  D  D  K  R  L  I  F  Z  L  T  W  E  P  Y
K  S  F  Z  L  T  Z  N  D  E  I  Z  E  T  M  J  M  X  L  S  G
H  T  J  G  T  R  P  E  D  H  R  C  F  L  U  K  H  X  P  G  T
Z  E  T  R  N  N  Y  N  P  L  T  M  V  K  Z  L  V  Y  M  N  M
C  R  N  R  K  A  Z  O  J  I  Q  D  A  W  T  F  G  D  O  I  R
R  O  X  N  L  N  N  R  O  K  N  V  T  T  M  W  N  G  C  S  N
K  I  V  E  B  I  G  N  K  K  B  Y  Q  X  I  K  Y  R  A  O  G
M  D  D  D  S  K  V  Y  L  D  H  C  F  K  B  T  N  B  R  L  C
P  S  K  O  L  G  V  C  M  C  B  M  C  C  R  R  I  Y  N  Y  R
T  N  E  Z  L  G  H  K  N  G  K  N  P  Q  R  F  Q  S  D  K  T
X  R  F  Y  Q  Y  N  T  T  G  F  Q  M  W  Q  B  L  G  P  N  T
L  R  F  P  W  M  M  F  C  Y  T  O  K  I  N  E  S  R  M  A  H
```

CLUES:
- When antigens clump.
- A nursing intervention for this disorder is a very firm mattress and no pillows when sleeping.
- A type I hypersensitivity that eventually leads to a thickening of the dermis with less sweat production in these areas.
- These are formed in type III hypersensitivity reactions, which then occlude blood vessels.
- These medications that are frequently used with immune system disorders should never be suddenly discontinued.
- Agents of the immune system that act to modify and enhance the immune and inflammatory responses.
- Type IV hypersensitivity reactions tend to be this—not immediate.
- These particular lymphocytes elevate in an allergic reaction as seen with type I hypersensitivities.
- The main complication for a patient with hypogammaglobulinemia.
- Another term for hives.

IMMUNE PUZZLE

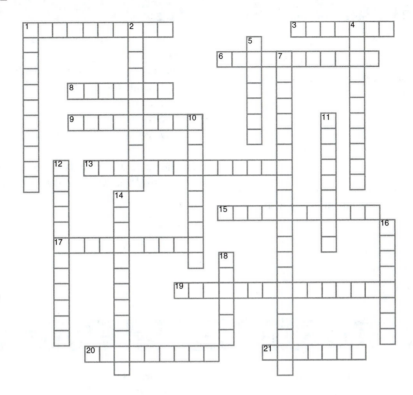

Across

1. A type of anemia that will develop in patients with autoimmune gastritis.
3. The number of minutes that a nurse should stay with a patient at the beginning of a blood transfusion.
6. This is a very serious type I hypersensitivity reaction.
8. An antibody-mediated response produced by B lymphocytes.
9. One of the causes of urticaria.
13. Hashimoto's thyroiditis begins with this effect.
15. These are a complication of repeated episodes of allergic rhinitis.
17. Similar to urticaria, although tends to be less pruritic, lasts longer, and involves deeper tissue.
19. The substance that is required in order for vitamin B_{12} to be absorbed in the small intestine.
20. Facial rash appearance in SLE patients.
21. This form of lupus erythematosus affects only the skin.

Down

1. Today, serum sickness tends to occur after administration of sulfonamides and these drugs.
2. A respiratory finding that is considered an emergency in a patient with angioedema.
4. Drug of choice during an anaphylactic reaction.
5. This can overwhelmingly affect the activities of daily living of a patient with SLE.
7. This disorder is due to defective functioning B cells.
10. One group of joints that is affected in ankylosing spondylitis.
11. IgE antibodies attach to these cells in a type I hypersensitivity reaction.
12. A significant type of contact dermatitis.
14. Ankylosing spondylitis is attributed to this.
16. A foreign protein or cell capable of causing an immune response.
18. An SLE flare trigger.

WORDS FOR IMMUNE PUZZLE

Allergen
Anaphylaxis
Angioedema
Autoimmunity
Butterfly
Discoid
Epinephrine
Fatigue

Fifteen
Humoral
Hypogammaglobulinemia
Hypothyroidism
Intrinsic factor
Latex allergy
Mast cells
Medicines

Nasal polyps
Obstruction
Penicillins
Pernicious
Sacroiliac
Stress

REVIEW QUESTIONS—CONTENT REVIEW

Choose the best answer unless directed otherwise.

1. As the nurse collects data on a patient, which of the following is a symptom the nurse would find for the patient with anaphylaxis?
   1. Dermatitis
   2. Delirium
   3. Sinusitis
   4. Wheezing

2. Which of the following is the medication of choice for anaphylaxis that the nurse should anticipate would be ordered?
   1. Epinephrine
   2. Theophylline (Theo-Dur)
   3. Digoxin (Lanoxin)
   4. Furosemide (Lasix)

3. Which of the following is a disease process characterized by a chronic progressive inflammation of the sacroiliac and costovertebral joints and adjacent soft tissue?
   1. Rheumatoid arthritis
   2. Kyphosis
   3. Scoliosis
   4. Ankylosing spondylitis

4. The nurse understands that an anaphylactic reaction is considered which of the following types of hypersensitivity reactions?
   1. Type I
   2. Type II
   3. Type III
   4. Type IV

REVIEW QUESTIONS—TEST PREPARATION

Choose the best answer unless directed otherwise.

5. In planning care for a patient who has allergic rhinitis, the nurse understands that without adherence to the treatment regimen, the patient is at risk for developing which of the following?
   1. Sinusitis
   2. Anaphylaxis
   3. Lymphadenopathy
   4. Angioedema

6. A patient reports on admission being "very sick" after taking erythromycin in the past. The patient is to receive erythromycin now. Which of the following actions should the nurse take first regarding the antibiotic?
   1. Give the antibiotic.
   2. Give half of the dose.
   3. Do not give the antibiotic.
   4. Discontinue the antibiotic.

7. A patient is being given penicillin via intravenous infusion and develops signs and symptoms of an anaphylactic reaction. Which of the following should be the nurse's first action?
   1. Call the doctor.
   2. Call for help.
   3. Maintain the antibiotic.
   4. Turn off the antibiotic.

8. A patient is admitted with a 2-month history of fatigue, shortness of breath, pallor, and dizziness. The patient is diagnosed with idiopathic autoimmune hemolytic anemia. On reviewing the laboratory results, the nurse notes the presence of which of the following which confirms this diagnosis?
   1. Red blood cell fragments
   2. Macrocytic, normochromic red blood cells
   3. Microcytic, hypochromic red blood cells
   4. Hemoglobin molecules

9. A portion of a patient's stomach was removed, so the patient is to take vitamin B_{12}. Which of the following statements should be included in the patient's teaching?
   1. "You will develop iron-deficiency anemia if you fail to take vitamin B_{12}."
   2. "Pernicious anemia is a complication of this surgery, so you need lifelong vitamin B_{12}."
   3. "Most patients who do not take vitamin B_{12} develop sickle cell anemia."
   4. "Taking vitamin B_{12} is important if you want to prevent acquired hemolytic anemia."

10. A patient is diagnosed with Hashimoto thyroiditis and asks what causes it. The nurse would respond that the destruction of thyroid cells in this condition is due to which of the following?
    1. Antigen–antibody complexes
    2. Autoantibodies
    3. Viral infection
    4. Bacterial infection

11. A patient who was walking in the woods disturbed a beehive, was stung two times, and was taken to the emergency department immediately due to allergies to bee stings. Which of the following symptoms would the nurse expect to see upon admission of this patient? **Select all that apply.**
    1. Pallor around the areas stung
    2. Numbness and tingling in the extremities
    3. Respiratory stridor
    4. Retinal hemorrhage
    5. Tachycardia
    6. Dyspnea

12. A patient has a long-standing history of allergies to pollen. Which of the following actions indicates that further teaching is necessary?
    1. The patient stays indoors on dry, windy days.
    2. The patient drives the car with the windows open.
    3. The patient avoids walking outside in the spring.
    4. The patient works in the garden on sunny days.

13. The nurse would evaluate that the patient understands what triggers allergic rhinitis by which of the following patient responses?
    1. "Injected medications."
    2. "Topical creams and ointments."
    3. "Ingested food and medications."
    4. "Airborne pollens and molds."

14. In collecting data for a patient with angioedema, the nurse understands how angioedema differs from urticaria because angioedema is characterized by which of the following?
    1. Angioedema has a deeper and more widespread edema.
    2. Angioedema has small, fluid-filled vesicles that crust.
    3. Angioedema lasts a shorter time.
    4. Angioedema is more pruritic.

15. Which of the following is a common nursing diagnosis that the nurse will include in the plan of care for a patient with systemic lupus erythematosus?
    1. *Fatigue*
    2. *Impaired Physical Mobility*
    3. *Impaired Swallowing*
    4. *Impaired Tissue Integrity*

16. The nurse is collecting data on a patient who has allergic rhinitis. Mark the area where the nurse would look for the presence of allergic shiners.

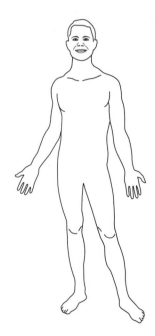

CHAPTER 20
Nursing Care of Patients With HIV Disease and AIDS

Name:	
Date:	
Course:	
Instructor:	

AUDIO CASE STUDY

Listen to the audio case study available on Davis Edge and then answer the following questions.

Mrs. Harris and HIV

1. For what age and ethnic groups is HIV increasing?

   _____
   _____
   _____
   _____
   _____

2. What are HIV sexual risk factors?

   _____
   _____
   _____
   _____
   _____

3. Can you get HIV/AIDS from kissing or hugging someone?

   _____
   _____
   _____
   _____
   _____

VOCABULARY

Fill in the blank.

1. _____ is the final phase of a chronic, progressive immune function disorder caused by HIV.

2. The _____ cell is an important part of the human immune system and helps defend the body against very primitive invaders such as fungi, yeast, and other viruses.

3. _____ is a diagnostic test done to measure resistance to currently available antiviral treatments.

4. _____ are a primary complication of HIV infection and occur because of an impaired immune system.

5. _____ occurs in some patients with AIDS and is characterized by an involuntary baseline body weight loss of more than 10%, with either weakness or fever for more than 30 days or chronic diarrhea of two loose stools daily for more than 30 days.

6. _____ measures the amount of HIV RNA in plasma and is extremely important for determining prognosis and monitoring the response to antiretroviral therapy.

DIAGNOSTIC TESTS

Describe the use of each of the following diagnostic tests.

1. HIV antigen/antibody combination immunoassay

_____
_____
_____
_____
_____

2. Viral load

_____
_____
_____
_____
_____

3. CD4 T lymphocyte count

_____
_____
_____
_____
_____

4. Genotyping

_____
_____
_____
_____
_____

HIV

Fill in the blanks.

1. HIV is transmitted through _____, _____, _____, and _____.

2. HIV may stay latent for _____ years.

3. Fatigue, headache, fever, and generalized lymphadenopathy may be seen during the _____ stage of HIV infection.

4. The time between HIV infection and developing HIV antibodies is called the _____ period.

HIV AND AIDS

Indicate whether the following are true or false, and correct false statements.

1. _____ If a health care worker is stuck with a needle from a patient with AIDS, exposure to the virus may occur even if gloves were worn.

2. _____ HIV is caused by AIDS.

3. _____ Individuals who are not men who have sex with men or who are not intravenous (IV) drug users do not need to worry about contracting HIV.

4. _____ If the nurse suctions a patient who is diagnosed with HIV and has a fresh tracheostomy and blood-tinged sputum gets in the nurse's eyes, the nurse may contract the virus.

5. _____ Once a person is infected with HIV, diagnosis can be made using laboratory tests within 1 to 2 days.

6. _____ A patient with AIDS should always be placed into isolation for the protection of health care workers.

CRITICAL THINKING

Answer the following questions.

1. Jack Swope, age 26, has been diagnosed as HIV positive. He asks, "Do I have AIDS, and am I going to die?" What should you say to him?

_____

_____

_____

_____

2. When is the patient with HIV considered to have developed AIDS?

_____

_____

_____

3. Jack is started on a combination of trimethoprim-sulfamethoxazole (TMP-SMX [Bactrim, Septra, Cotrim]) medication. Why?

_____

_____

_____

4. Later, Jack is diagnosed with AIDS with a CD4 T lymphocyte count of 200 cells/microL.

(a) Jack is 6 feet tall and weighs 135 lb. He is malnourished. What are possible reasons? _____

_____

_____

_____

_____

_____

(b) What can you do as a nurse to improve Jack's nutrition?

_____

_____

_____

_____

_____

5. Six months after being diagnosed with AIDS, Jack develops dementia. Why?

_____

_____

_____

_____

_____

_____

_____

6. How can a nurse contract HIV from a patient?

_____

_____

_____

_____

_____

7. How should the home health care nurse teach family members of a patient with AIDS to clean the patient's home?

_____

_____

_____

_____

_____

_____

REVIEW QUESTIONS—CONTENT REVIEW

Choose the best answer unless directed otherwise.

1. Which of the following best defines AIDS?
   1. AIDS is a syndrome that always develops after infection with HIV.
   2. AIDS is the final phase of a chronic progressive immune disorder caused by HIV.
   3. AIDS is characterized by a CD4 T lymphocyte count greater than 14% of total lymphocytes.
   4. AIDS is an acute reversible syndrome.

2. For HIV-infected patients being prescribed antiretroviral therapy who have consistent CD4 lymphocyte counts levels above 300 cells/microL and suppressed viral load testing, when is CD4 T lymphocyte testing recommended to be done? **Select all that apply.**
   1. Before antiretroviral therapy
   2. Every month
   3. At 3 months
   4. Every 2 months during antiretroviral therapy
   5. Every 3 to 6 months for 2 years
   6. Annually after 2 years

REVIEW QUESTIONS—TEST PREPARATION

Choose the best answer unless directed otherwise.

3. In planning an educational session for a patient with HIV, the nurse would include that contact with which of the following body fluids can transmit HIV? **Select all that apply.**
   1. Saliva
   2. Tears
   3. Breast milk
   4. Semen
   5. Blood
   6. Sweat

4. A patient who is being tested for HIV asks what types of tests are used. Which of the following tests would the nurse state can be used to identify an HIV infection? **Select all that apply.**
   1. CD4 T lymphocyte count
   2. Genotyping
   3. HIV antibody/antigen combination immunoassay
   4. Nucleic acid test
   5. Urinalysis

5. The nurse is caring for a patient with HIV who has diarrhea. Which of the following would be most therapeutic to teach the patient to avoid in the diet to reduce diarrhea?
   1. Potassium-rich foods
   2. High fiber diet
   3. Liquid nutritional supplements
   4. Frozen food products

6. The nurse is teaching a patient newly diagnosed with AIDS about complications of the disease. Which of the following is a more common opportunistic infection in AIDS?
   1. Candidiasis
   2. Kaposi sarcoma
   3. Mycoplasma pneumonia
   4. Toxoplasmosis

7. The nurse is taking vital signs of a pregnant woman during her first prenatal visit. The patient asks the nurse if she has to have an HIV test. Which of the following is the nurse's best response?
   1. "Yes, all pregnant women must have an HIV test in their third trimester."
   2. "If you do not have multiple sex partners or inject drugs, it is not necessary."
   3. "Governmental guidelines require an HIV test for all pregnant woman."
   4. "After pretest counseling, you decide whether HIV testing should be done."

8. The nurse is caring for a patient with HIV. Which of the following foods would the nurse teach the patient are safe to eat to reduce the risk of an infection? **Select all that apply.**
   1. Caesar dressing
   2. Cooked vegetables
   3. Feta cheese
   4. Raw fruits
   5. Raw vegetables
   6. Self-peeled fruits

9. When caring for a patient with AIDS, which of the following actions should the nurse take for infection control?
   1. Wear gloves at all times.
   2. Wear gloves for blood/body fluid contact.
   3. Wear gown and mask at all times.
   4. Wear a mask during patient contact times.

10. The nurse is reinforcing teaching on the frequency of viral load testing for a patient who has HIV and is to begin antiretroviral therapy. Which of the following general viral load testing recommendations, for those with consistently suppressed viral loads on antiretroviral therapy, would the nurse include?
    Select all that apply.
    1. Before antiretroviral therapy
    2. On day 1 of antiretroviral therapy
    3. Within 1 month
    4. Every 2 months during antiretroviral therapy
    5. Every 3 to 4 months for 2 years
    6. Every 6 months after 2 years

11. The nurse is providing HIV risk–reduction reinforcement for a patient who is 55 years old. Which of the following information should the nurse include?
    Select all that apply.
    1. Anal, oral, and vaginal sexual activity requires a latex barrier be used.
    2. Condoms are needed only when a person discloses being HIV positive.
    3. Having a sexually transmitted infection increases the risk of acquiring HIV.
    4. A new condom is needed for each sexual activity.
    5. Petroleum jelly can be used as a lubricant during condom use.
    6. Condoms are only useful for birth control.

CHAPTER 21
Cardiovascular System Function, Assessment, and Therapeutic Measures

Name:	_____
Date:	_____
Course:	_____
Instructor:	_____

AUDIO CASE STUDY

Listen to the audio case study available on Davis Edge and then answer the following questions.

Mr. Flores Is Undergoing a Cardiac Catheterization

1. In what ways does the nurse prepare Mr. Flores prior to the procedure?

   _____

   _____

   _____

   _____

2. During cardiac catheterization, what cardiopulmonary measurements can be obtained?

   _____

   _____

3. What preprocedure instructions was Mr. Flores given?

   _____

   _____

   _____

   _____

STRUCTURES OF THE CARDIOVASCULAR SYSTEM

Label the following structures.

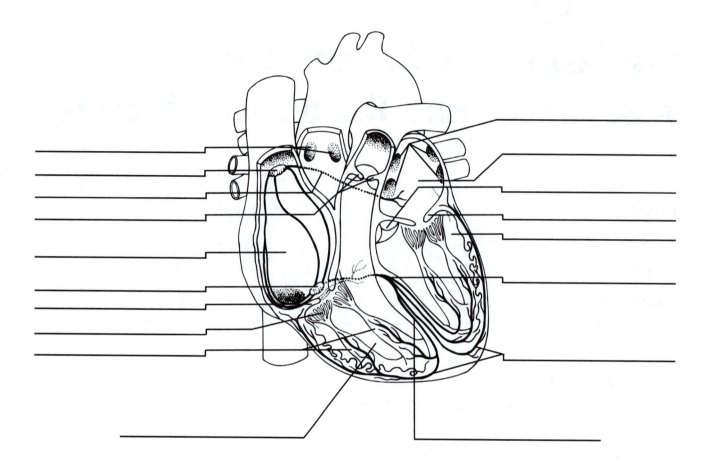

CARDIAC BLOOD FLOW

Number the following in proper sequence with respect to the flow of blood through the heart and to and from the lungs and body. Begin with the caval veins.

1. _____ Superior and inferior caval veins
2. _____ Left ventricle
3. _____ Right atrium
4. _____ Right ventricle
5. _____ Body
6. _____ Lungs
7. _____ Pulmonary artery
8. _____ Pulmonary veins
9. _____ Aorta
10. _____ Left atrium
11. _____ Mitral valve
12. _____ Aortic valve
13. _____ Tricuspid valve
14. _____ Pulmonic valve

AGING AND THE CARDIOVASCULAR SYSTEM

Find the 11 errors and insert the correct information.

It is believed that the "aging" of blood vessels, especially

arteries, begins in adulthood. Average resting blood pressure

tends to decrease with age and may contribute to stroke or

right-sided heart failure. The thicker walled veins, especially

those of the legs, may also weaken and stretch, making their

valves incompetent.

With age, the heart lining becomes less efficient, and there is an increase in both maximum cardiac output and heart rate. The health of the myocardium depends on the lungs' blood supply. Hypertension causes the right ventricle to work harder, so it may atrophy. The heart valves may become thinner from fibrosis, leading to heart murmurs. Arrhythmias become more common in older adults as the cells of the conduction pathway become more efficient.

CARDIOVASCULAR SYSTEM

Fill in the blanks.

1. The function of the _____ system is to carry oxygen and nutrients to the tissues and remove waste products.

2. The _____ function is to pump blood.

3. The peripheral _____ system is composed of arteries, veins, _____, and lymph vessels.

4. With aging, the walls of blood vessels _____.

5. The heart sound _____ occurs at the beginning of systole, when the atrioventricular valves close, and the sound *dub* occurs at the start of _____, when the semilunar valves close.

6. Palpation of pulse quality is recorded as _____ 0; weak, thready 1+; _____ 2+; bounding 3+.

7. Tests to assess _____ function may include x-rays, electrocardiogram (ECG), exercise stress test, echocardiogram, thallium scan, dipyridamole thallium scan, multiple gated acquisition, serum troponin I, creatine kinase (CK), CK-MB, myoglobin, cardiac _____, and angiography.

8. The six Ps characterize _____ vascular disease: _____, _____, pallor, pulselessness, paralysis, and _____.

9. Tests to assess peripheral _____ disease include Doppler ultrasound, peripheral vascular stress testing, _____, and arteriography.

10. _____ is an amino acid in the blood that may damage the lining of arteries and promote blood clots, which increases cardiovascular disease risk.

ACUTE CARDIOVASCULAR DATA COLLECTION

Identify the word that is obtained during a history for the description given.

1. _____ Checked before administration of medications and diagnostic dyes

2. _____ Modifiable risk factor for cardiovascular disorders that is a habit

3. _____ Location: chest, calf; radiation: arms, jaw, neck

4. _____ Sign resulting from right-sided heart failure

5. _____ Lung sounds heard with left-sided heart failure

6. _____ Symptom with an arrhythmia

7. _____ An effect of having decreased cardiac output

8. _____ Classic sign of acute heart failure (pulmonary edema)

9. _____ Normally 3 seconds or less

10. _____ Distal ends of fingers swollen and clublike

CRITICAL THINKING

Make a concept map for a patient who is to undergo a cardiac catheterization. A concept map can help you visualize the patient's needs. Think of possible categories of needs of this patient and then complete activities and needs under each category. Some categories have been given to get you started, but include others you think of. You can get even more detailed and create subcategories for each activity or need.

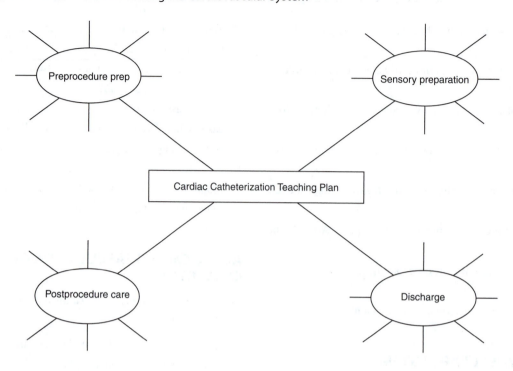

REVIEW QUESTIONS—CONTENT REVIEW

Choose the best answer unless directed otherwise.

1. Each normal heartbeat is initiated by which of the following?
   1. Cardiac center in the medulla
   2. Bundle of His in the interventricular septum
   3. Sinoatrial node in the wall of the right atrium
   4. Sympathetic nerves from the spinal cord

2. During one cardiac cycle, which of the following occurs?
   1. Ventricles contract first, followed by the atria.
   2. Atria and ventricles contract simultaneously.
   3. Atria contract first, followed by the ventricles.
   4. Ventricles contract twice for every contraction of the atria.

3. Which of the following detects changes in blood pressure?
   1. Pressoreceptors in the medulla
   2. Blood vessels in the medulla
   3. Coronary vessels in the myocardium
   4. Pressoreceptors in the carotid and aortic sinuses

4. Epinephrine increases blood pressure because it does which of the following?
   1. Increases water resorption by the kidneys
   2. Increases heart rate and force of cardiac contraction
   3. Causes vasodilation in the skin and viscera
   4. Decreases heart rate and force of contraction

5. When blood pressure decreases, the kidneys help raise it by secreting which of the following?
   1. Renin
   2. Epinephrine
   3. Aldosterone
   4. Erythropoietin

6. Which of the following prevents the backflow of blood in veins?
   1. Middle layer of vein
   2. Precapillary sphincters
   3. Smooth muscles
   4. Valves

7. The tricuspid and mitral valves prevent backflow of blood from which of the following?
   1. Ventricles to atria when the ventricles contract
   2. Atria to ventricles when the ventricles relax
   3. Ventricles to atria when the atria contract
   4. Atria to ventricles when the atria contract

8. Which of the following describes the purpose of the endocardium of the heart?
   1. Covers the heart muscle and prevents friction.
   2. Supports the coronary blood vessels.
   3. Lines the chambers of the heart and prevents abnormal clotting.
   4. Prevents backflow of blood from atria to ventricles.

9. Which of the following is the function of the coronary arteries?
   1. To carry deoxygenated blood to the myocardium
   2. To carry oxygenated blood to the myocardium
   3. To carry deoxygenated blood to the lungs
   4. To carry oxygenated blood to the lungs

10. Where in the nervous system is the cardiac center found?
    1. Cerebrum
    2. Hypothalamus
    3. Medulla
    4. Spinal cord

11. Angiotensin II causes which of the following?
    1. Vasodilation and antidiuretic hormone (ADH) secretion
    2. Vasoconstriction and aldosterone secretion
    3. Increased heart rate and vasodilation
    4. Increased heart rate and ADH secretion

12. The increase of resting blood pressure with age may contribute to which of the following?
    1. Arrhythmias
    2. Left-sided heart failure
    3. Peripheral edema
    4. Thrombus formation

REVIEW QUESTIONS—TEST PREPARATION

Choose the best answer unless directed otherwise.

13. A patient had a bilateral mastectomy 2 days ago, so the nurse obtains blood pressure readings from the patient's legs. The patient's baseline blood pressure in the arm was 112/78 mm Hg. Which of the following readings, when compared with baseline blood pressure, does the nurse expect when taking the blood pressure in the leg?
    1. 122/84 mm Hg
    2. 102/68 mm Hg
    3. 100/78 mm Hg
    4. 96/58 mm Hg

14. The nurse obtains a lower blood pressure reading on a patient's left arm than the right arm. As a result, which of the following extremities would the nurse use for ongoing blood pressure measurement?
    1. Left arm
    2. Right arm
    3. Right leg
    4. Either arm

15. The nurse is checking a patient's blood pressure for orthostatic hypotension. The patient's blood pressure was 142/88 mm Hg when lying down and 136/80 mm Hg when standing. The patient asks the nurse why there is such a difference. Which of the following is the best response by the nurse?
    1. "Your blood pressure should have gone up about 5 mm Hg, so we'll need to have you move very slowly to avoid a fall."
    2. "Blood pressure usually compensates for a change in position by going down by about 15 mm Hg, so this is normal."
    3. "It is safe for the blood pressure to drop by as much as 25 mm Hg, so you don't need to worry."
    4. "Your blood pressure is still in a normal range, so there is no real concern."

16. The nurse obtains a pulse of 78 beats per minute and a lying blood pressure of 122/76 mm Hg on a patient. When the nurse checks the patient's blood pressure for orthostatic hypotension, the patient's heart rate is 92 beats per minute, and the blood pressure is 116/68 mm Hg. Which of the following actions should the nurse take?
    1. Return the patient to a lying position immediately.
    2. Ask if the patient is experiencing chest pain.
    3. Document that normal compensation occurred.
    4. Document that orthostatic hypotension is present.

17. The nurse is inspecting a patient's legs during data collection and notes that there is bilateral decreased hair distribution; long, thick, brittle nails; and shiny, taut, dry skin. The nurse understands that this can indicate which of the following? Which action would the nurse avoid performing based on these data?
    1. Positioning the legs dependently
    2. Elevating the legs
    3. Applying lotion to the legs
    4. Filing toenails

18. The nurse is explaining to a patient that for a thallium stress test, dipyridamole (Persantine), a coronary vasodilator, will be given. Which of the following would the nurse include in the teaching regarding the reason this medication is being given?
    1. To decrease cardiac output
    2. To increase cardiac blood flow like exercise would
    3. To prevent a clot from forming during the test
    4. To reduce systemic vascular resistance

19. Which of the following data would be most important for the nurse to collect immediately for a patient who is reporting fatigue and dizziness? **Select all that apply.**
    1. Presence of pain
    2. Capillary refill
    3. Vital signs
    4. Presence of dyspnea
    5. White blood cell count
    6. Heart rhythm

20. The nurse would evaluate the patient as understanding teaching for a cardiac catheterization if the patient stated which of the following? **Select all that apply.**
    1. "I will be awake during the test."
    2. "It will take 1 hour."
    3. "I will be on a stationary bed."
    4. "The dye can cause a warm sensation."
    5. "There will be a lot of equipment in the room."
    6. "My heart will be monitored constantly."

21. The nurse is collecting data on a patient with a diagnosis of right-sided heart failure. Mark the area of the finding that supports this diagnosis.

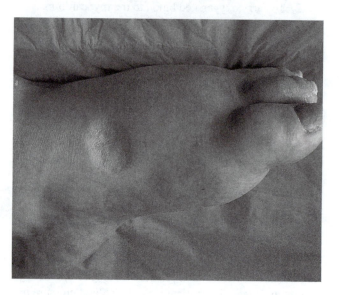

CHAPTER 22
Nursing Care of Patients With Hypertension

Name:	_____
Date:	_____
Course:	_____
Instructor:	_____

AUDIO CASE STUDY

Listen to the audio case study available on Davis Edge and then answer the following questions.

Jenice and Hypertension

1. What actions does Jenice take to ensure an accurate blood pressure (BP) is obtained?

   _____

   _____

   _____

   _____

   _____

2. What does the patient's obtained BP of 118/70 mm Hg indicate?

   _____

   _____

   _____

   _____

   _____

3. What actions are taken for the patient with a BP of 196/94 mm Hg?

   _____

   _____

   _____

   _____

   _____

VOCABULARY

Match the word with its definition.

1. _____ Atherosclerosis
2. _____ Peripheral vascular resistance
3. _____ Hypertension
4. _____ Diastolic BP
5. _____ Cardiac output
6. _____ Systolic BP
7. _____ Secondary hypertension
8. _____ Primary hypertension

1. Amount of blood the heart pumps out each minute
2. Most common form of arteriosclerosis, in which fats are deposited on arterial walls
3. Amount of pressure exerted on the wall of the arteries when the ventricles are at rest; the bottom number in a BP reading
4. Abnormally elevated BP
5. Opposition to blood flow through the vessels
6. Abnormally elevated BP, the cause of which is unknown; also called *essential hypertension*
7. Maximal pressure exerted on the arteries during contraction of the left ventricle of the heart; top number of a BP reading
8. High BP that is a symptom of a specific cause, such as a kidney abnormality

DIURETICS

Select the number that identifies the type of each diuretic.

1. _____ spironolactone (Aldactone)
2. _____ bumetanide (Bumex)
3. _____ chlorothiazide (Diuril)
4. _____ torsemide (Demadex)
5. _____ furosemide (Lasix)
6. _____ amiloride (Midamor)
7. _____ metolazone (Zaroxolyn)
8. _____ hydrochlorothiazide (HydroDIURIL)

1. Thiazide or thiazide-like
2. Loop
3. Potassium-sparing

HYPERTENSION RISK FACTORS

Indicate whether the statement is true or false.

1. _____ Increased stress can be a cause of hypertension.
2. _____ There is a link between a high-fat diet, obesity, and hypertension.
3. _____ High calcium, potassium, and magnesium levels are important risk factors for the development of hypertension.
4. _____ People who are not active on a regular basis are at an increased risk of developing hypertension.
5. _____ A diet high in salt is also high in vitamins and minerals.
6. _____ Inadequate sleep of less than 5 hours is a risk factor for hypertension.
7. _____ Classical music for 30 minutes daily can reduce BP.

BLOOD PRESSURE CATEGORIES

Identify the category of the blood pressure measurement.

1. _____ BP 124/72 mm Hg
2. _____ BP 110/68 mm Hg
3. _____ BP 134/94 mm Hg
4. _____ BP 126/78 mm Hg
5. _____ BP 130/80 mm Hg

CRITICAL THINKING

Read the following case study and answer the questions.

Mrs. Laura Martin, age 42, is seen in the hypertension clinic for a follow-up visit for hypertension. Her BP is 160/92 mm Hg, and she is diagnosed with hypertension. The health care provider encourages continued lifestyle modification and prescribes hydrochlorothiazide (HydroDIURIL).

1. Why is hydrochlorothiazide prescribed? _____
_____
_____
_____

2. What additional information should the nurse collect to develop a teaching plan for lifestyle modifications and the medication? _____
_____
_____
_____
_____

3. Develop a teaching plan for Mrs. Martin's needs based on the data collected. _____
_____
_____
_____
_____

4. What interventions will help Mrs. Martin reach her goal for controlling her hypertension? _____
_____
_____
_____
_____

5. How will you know when Mrs. Martin has reached her goals? _____
_____
_____
_____
_____

REVIEW QUESTIONS—CONTENT REVIEW

Choose the best answer unless directed otherwise.

1. The nurse defines a normal blood pressure during a patient teaching session as which of these?
   1. Systolic lower than 120 mm Hg and diastolic lower than 80 mm Hg
   2. Systolic of 120 to 129 mm Hg and diastolic lower than 80 mm Hg
   3. Systolic of 130 to 139 mm Hg or diastolic of 80 to 89 mm Hg
   4. Systolic of 140 mm Hg or higher or diastolic of 90 mm Hg or higher

2. The nurse explains to a patient with blood pressure readings of 164/102 mm Hg and 176/100 mm Hg on two separate occasions that this type of hypertension is classified in which hypertension category?
   1. Elevated
   2. Stage 1
   3. Stage 2

REVIEW QUESTIONS—TEST PREPARATION

Choose the best answer unless directed otherwise.

3. The nurse would evaluate the patient as understanding the teaching of the action of enalapril maleate (Vasotec) if the patient stated which of these?
   1. "Vasotec decreases levels of angiotensin II."
   2. "Vasotec increases heart rate."
   3. "Vasotec dilates the arterioles and veins."
   4. "Vasotec decreases cardiac output."

4. The nurse would include which of the following to describe the action of diltiazem (Cardizem) in the patient's teaching plan?
   1. It increases heart rate.
   2. It vasodilates.
   3. It decreases fluid volume.
   4. It increases cardiac contractility.

5. The nurse is developing a teaching plan for a patient. Which of the following should the nurse include as a modifiable risk factor for the development of hypertension? **Select all that apply.**
   1. Race
   2. High cholesterol
   3. Cigarette smoking
   4. Sedentary lifestyle
   5. Less than 5 hours of sleep

6. The patient asks the nurse, "How is stage 2 hypertension defined?" Which of the following is the best response by the nurse?
   1. "It is a measurement of the heart's cardiac output as blood is pumped into the aorta."
   2. "It is a systolic of at least 140 mm Hg or a diastolic of at least 90 mm Hg averaged on two occasions."
   3. "It is hypertension that is regulated by stress, activity, and emotions."
   4. "It is a systolic of 130 mm Hg or a diastolic of 80 mm Hg averaged on two occasions."

7. The nurse is developing a teaching plan to help a patient control hypertension. The teaching plan should include which of the following lifestyle modifications?
   1. Regular aerobic exercise
   2. Low-tar cigarettes
   3. Three alcoholic beverages per day
   4. Daily multivitamin supplements

8. A patient calls the hypertension clinic to report frequent headaches after taking a newly prescribed medication. The nurse anticipates that this is an expected side effect if the patient is taking which of the following medications?
   1. Furosemide (Lasix)
   2. Atenolol (Tenormin)
   3. Clonidine (Catapres)
   4. Hydralazine (Apresoline)

9. A patient has been prescribed bumetanide (Bumex) daily to control hypertension. Which of the following patient statements indicates correct knowledge of the treatment regimen?
   1. "I can go to the beach and play in the sun all day."
   2. "Now I can eat whatever I want, whenever I want."
   3. "I'll take my medication when I get up in the morning."
   4. "I won't need any medication once my blood pressure goes down."

10. Which common side effect of metolazone (Zaroxolyn) should the nurse instruct a patient to report to the health care provider?
    1. Numb hands
    2. Muscle weakness
    3. Gastrointestinal distress
    4. Nightmares

11. The nurse understands that which of the following is a side effect most likely to be reported by patients receiving enalapril maleate (Vasotec)?
    1. Acne
    2. Cough
    3. Diarrhea
    4. Heartburn

12. What action should the nurse take before administering diltiazem (Cardizem) for hypertension?
    1. Check calcium level.
    2. Ask patient if appetite has changed.
    3. Obtain vital signs.
    4. Inform patient not to stop medication abruptly.

13. Which of the following nursing diagnoses is the focus of care for a patient with hypertension?
    1. *Activity Intolerance*
    2. *Ineffective Airway Clearance*
    3. *Impaired Physical Mobility*
    4. *Readiness for Enhanced Health Literacy*

14. Which of the following statements, if made by a patient with hypertension, indicates to the nurse a need for more teaching? **Select all that apply.**
    1. "Hypertension may damage the kidneys and eyes."
    2. "I will limit my salt intake."
    3. "Medication will no longer be needed when I feel better."
    4. "People often do not know when their blood pressure is high."
    5. "Hypertension can be cured."

15. The nurse would evaluate amlodipine (Norvasc) as being effective if which of these blood pressures readings were obtained?
    1. 88/52 mm Hg
    2. 118/70 mm Hg
    3. 138/82 mm Hg
    4. 142/86 mm Hg

CHAPTER 23

Nursing Care of Patients With Valvular, Inflammatory, and Infectious Cardiac or Venous Disorders

Name: _____	
Date: _____	
Course: _____	
Instructor: _____	

AUDIO CASE STUDY

Listen to the audio case study available on Davis Edge and then answer the following questions.

Mrs. Bell: Mitral Regurgitation and Anticoagulants

1. What symptoms of mitral regurgitation is Mrs. Bell having?

   _____
   _____
   _____
   _____

2. What do diagnostic tests reveal for Mrs. Bell?

   _____
   _____
   _____
   _____
   _____

3. What occurs in mitral regurgitation?

   _____
   _____
   _____
   _____
   _____

4. What safety precautions are taught to Mrs. Bell for the anticoagulants she is to take?

_____

_____

_____

_____

_____

_____

VOCABULARY

Fill in the blank with the word that is formed by the word building.

1. _____ annulus (ring) + plasty (formed)
2. _____ commissura (joining together) + tome (incision)
3. _____ in (not) + sufficiens (sufficient)
4. _____ re (again) + gurgitare (to flood)
5. _____ stenos (narrow)
6. _____ valvula (leaf of a folding door) + plasty (formed)
7. _____ choreia (dance)
8. _____ peri (around) + kardia (heart) + itis (inflammation)
9. _____ myo (muscle) + kardia (heart) + itis (inflammation)
10. _____ petecchia (skin spot)
11. _____ peri (around) + kardia (heart) + kentesis (puncture)
12. _____ kardia (heart) + tamponade (plug)
13. _____ kardia (heart) + myo (muscle) + pathy (disease)
14. _____ kardia (heart) + mega (large)
15. _____ my (muscle) + ectomy (cutting out)
16. _____ thromb (lump [clot]) + phleb (vein) + itis (inflammation)

MITRAL VALVE PROLAPSE

Find the eight errors and insert the correct information.

During ventricular diastole, when pressures in the left ventricle rise, the leaflets of the mitral valve normally remain open. In mitral valve prolapse (MVP), however, the leaflets bulge backward into the left ventricle during systole. Often there are functional problems seen with MVP. However, if the leaflets do not fit together, mitral stenosis can occur with varying degrees of severity.

MVP tends to be hereditary, and the cause is known. Infections that damage the mitral valve may be a contributing factor. It is the most common form of valvular heart disease and typically occurs in men aged 20 to 55. Most patients with MVP have symptoms. Symptoms that may occur include chest pain, arrhythmias, palpitations, dizziness, and syncope. No treatment is needed unless symptoms are present. Stimulants and caffeine should be avoided to prevent symptoms.

VALVULAR DISORDERS

Indicate whether the statement is true or false, and correct false statements.

1. _____ Stenosis is widening of the opening of a heart valve.

2. _____ Stenosis inhibits the forward flow of blood.

3. _____ Regurgitation, or insufficiency, is failure of the valve to close completely.

4. _____ Regurgitation inhibits backflow of blood.

5. _____ Rheumatic heart disease and congenital defects are primary causes of valvular disease.

6. _____ The primary valves affected by disease are the tricuspid and pulmonic valves.

7. _____ Compensatory mechanisms in valvular disease are dilation to handle the increased blood volume and hypertrophy to increase the strength of contractions.

8. _____ Symptoms of valvular disease often occur early and reflect decreased cardiac output and pulmonary congestion (fatigue, dyspnea, orthopnea, cough).

9. _____ In severe valvular disease, heart failure occurs, and symptoms reflect the backup of blood from the failing chamber.

10. _____ In acute valve disorders, symptoms of shock are seen.

11. _____ Valve disease diagnosis is made with electrocardiogram, chest x-ray examination, echocardiogram, and cardiac catheterization.

12. _____ Valvuloplasty uses a balloon to separate the valve leaflets.

13. _____ Commissurotomy narrows the valve opening.

14. _____ Annuloplasty surgically repairs the valve.

15. _____ Patient teaching for valvular disorders includes understanding the importance of prophylactic antibiotics before all invasive procedures.

CRITICAL THINKING—MRS. MURPHY

Read the case study and answer the questions.

Mrs. Murphy, age 72, has aortic stenosis and is scheduled for an aortic valve replacement. She reports fatigue and dyspnea with exertion.

1. What may be the cause of Mrs. Murphy's aortic stenosis?

_____

_____

2. When obtaining Mrs. Murphy's medical history, what should the nurse ask that is relevant to the cause of aortic stenosis?

_____

_____

3. How does the heart compensate for aortic stenosis?

_____

_____

4. What should the nurse anticipate may occur in severe aortic stenosis?

_____

_____

5. Why is angina a common symptom of aortic stenosis?

_____

_____

_____

6. Mrs. Murphy's chest x-ray shows an enlarged heart. She asks the nurse why it is enlarged. How should the nurse explain this to Mrs. Murphy?

_____

_____

_____

_____

_____

7. Why is aortic stenosis treated with valvular replacement?

_____

_____

INFLAMMATORY AND INFECTIOUS CARDIOVASCULAR DISORDERS

Match the word with its definition.

1. _____ Vein may feel like a cord.
2. _____ Sac surrounding the heart is inflamed.
3. _____ Inflammation of the heart lining caused by microorganisms.
4. _____ Solid, liquid, gaseous masses of undissolved matter traveling with the current in a blood or lymphatic vessel.
5. _____ Severe damage to the heart from rheumatic fever.

1. Induration with superficial vein thrombophlebitis
2. Emboli
3. Infective endocarditis
4. Pericarditis
5. Rheumatic heart disease

RHEUMATIC FEVER AND RHEUMATIC HEART DISEASE

Find the six errors and insert the correct information.

Rheumatic fever causes a streptococcal infection such as a sore throat. Rheumatic fever signs and symptoms include polyarthritis, subcutaneous nodules, cholera with rapid and controlled movements, carditis, fever, arthralgia, and pneumonia. A throat culture diagnoses rheumatic fever. The heart valves and their structures can be scarred and damaged. Rheumatic fever can be prevented by detecting and treating streptococcal infections promptly with aspirin.

DIAGNOSTIC TESTS FOR INFECTIVE ENDOCARDITIS

Match the test with its finding that is indicative of infective endocarditis.

Test

1. _____ White blood cell count
2. _____ Blood cultures
3. _____ Electrocardiogram (ECG)
4. _____ Chest x-ray examination
5. _____ Echocardiogram

Finding

1. Vegetations on heart valves
2. Arrhythmias
3. Slight elevation
4. Heart failure
5. Identifies causative organism

THROMBOPHLEBITIS

Complete the rationale and evaluation of the nursing care plan for a patient with thrombophlebitis.

NURSING DIAGNOSIS
Acute Pain *related to inflammation of vein*

Intervention	Rationale	Evaluation
Monitor pain using a rating scale, such as 0 to 10.		
Provide analgesics and NSAIDs as ordered.		
Apply warm, moist compresses as ordered.		

NURSING DIAGNOSIS
Impaired Skin Integrity *related to venous stasis*

Intervention	Rationale	Evaluation
Observe skin for edema, skin color changes, and ulcers. Measure both extremities' circumference at the same site in each extremity daily or as ordered.		
Elevate feet above heart level.		
Fit and apply elastic compression stockings after edema is reduced, as ordered.		
Teach patient to avoid crossing legs or wearing constrictive clothes.		

CRITICAL THINKING—MR. EVANS

Read the case study and answer the questions.

Mr. Evans, age 68, is admitted to the hospital for heart failure resulting from hypertrophic cardiomyopathy. He has dyspnea, fatigue, and angina. His lung sounds reveal crackles.

1. What is the pathophysiology of hypertrophic cardiomyopathy? _____

_____

_____

2. What occurs in hypertrophic cardiomyopathy to ventricular size and ventricular filling with blood? _____

_____

_____

3. What diagnostic test will show hypertrophic cardiomyopathy and left-sided heart failure? _____

_____

_____

4. Why is digoxin (Lanoxin) contraindicated for Mr. Evans?

_____

_____

5. Why should Mr. Evans be taught to avoid (a) dehydration and (b) exertion? _____

_____

_____

_____

6. Why is it important for Mr. Evans's family to learn cardiopulmonary resuscitation (CPR)? _____

_____

_____

_____

CRITICAL THINKING—MRS. STRECKER

Read the case study and answer the questions.

Mrs. Strecker, an active 27-year-old accountant, has come into your clinic with reports of right leg pain, redness, and edema. During data collection, she reports being a cigarette smoker, having a sedentary job, eating two healthy meals daily, and exercising three times weekly. She states she takes a multivitamin daily and oral contraceptives. She is married with one child. Mrs. Strecker is diagnosed with deep vein thrombosis.

1. Which of the following nursing actions would be appropriate for Mrs. Strecker's plan of care?
   1. Encouraging early ambulation
   2. Teaching coughing and deep breathing
   3. Massaging lotion on both legs and feet to increase comfort
   4. Measuring the circumference of both legs at the same location

2. In developing a teaching plan for Mrs. Strecker, the nurse must identify risk factors for thrombophlebitis to be avoided upon recovery. Select all known risk factors for Mrs. Strecker in the development of thrombophlebitis.
   1. Exercise
   2. Sedentary job
   3. Taking multivitamins
   4. Eating habits
   5. Demanding job
   6. Cigarette smoking
   7. Oral contraceptives

3. Upon discharge, Mrs. Strecker asks what she can do to prevent a future occurrence of deep vein thrombosis. Which of these should the nurse teach Mrs. Strecker to help prevent deep vein thrombosis? **Select all that apply.**
   1. Take multivitamins
   2. Avoid exercise that may cause trauma
   3. Manage stress
   4. Avoid extended periods of sitting or standing
   5. Maintain adequate hydration

REVIEW QUESTIONS—CONTENT REVIEW

Choose the best answer unless directed otherwise.

1. Which of the following does the nurse understand occurs in aortic stenosis?
   1. Aortic valve does not close tightly.
   2. Emptying of blood from left ventricle is impaired.
   3. Blood backflows into the left atrium.
   4. Emptying of the left atrium is impaired.

2. The nurse understands that which of the following occurs in mitral regurgitation?
   1. Backflow of blood into the left atrium
   2. Backflow of blood into the right atrium
   3. Impaired emptying of the right ventricle
   4. Impaired emptying of the left ventricle

3. Which of the following compensatory mechanisms does the nurse understand occurs with ventricular valve disorders?
   1. Decreased atrial kick
   2. Atrial hypertrophy
   3. Ventricular hypertrophy
   4. Systolic hypertension

4. Which of the following does the nurse understand causes fatigue in patients with chronic aortic stenosis?
   1. Atrial fibrillation
   2. Left ventricular failure
   3. Decreased pulmonary blood flow
   4. Increased coronary artery blood flow

5. Which of the following diagnostic tests does the nurse understand measures the pressures in the cardiac chambers?
   1. Electrocardiogram
   2. Exercise stress test
   3. Echocardiogram
   4. Cardiac catheterization

6. Which of the following does the nurse understand usually precedes rheumatic fever?
   1. A viral infection
   2. A fungal infection
   3. A staphylococcal infection
   4. A beta-hemolytic streptococcal infection

7. During data collection, which of the following is the most common symptom of pericarditis that the nurse would expect to identify?
   1. Dyspnea
   2. Intermittent claudication
   3. Chest pain
   4. Calf pain

REVIEW QUESTIONS—TEST PREPARATION

Choose the best answer unless directed otherwise.

8. Which of the following should the nurse include in the plan of care as a patient outcome for *Deficient Knowledge* related to mitral stenosis?
   1. Patient will have clear breath sounds, no edema or weight gain
   2. Patient will exhibit less fatigue during self-care
   3. Patient will verbalize knowledge of disorder
   4. Patient will state fear is reduced

9. Which of the following medications does the nurse anticipate that the patient will be given to prevent complications associated with heart failure and decreased cardiac output? **Select all that apply.**
   1. Furosemide (Lasix)
   2. Cephalexin (Keflex)
   3. Penicillin (Bicillin)
   4. Prednisone (Deltasone)
   5. Reteplase or rPA (Retavase)
   6. Potassium supplement

10. The nurse is caring for a patient, age 75, who has a nursing diagnosis of *Deficient Knowledge* related to furosemide (Lasix) administration. Which of the following interventions is most essential to include when planning a teaching session?
    1. Determine patient's and family's learning priorities.
    2. Tell patient what must be learned first about furosemide.
    3. Determine patient's dietary intake of potassium.
    4. Give patient a written test at the end of the teaching session.

11. A patient, age 65, is being discharged after a mechanical valve replacement for aortic stenosis. Which of the following should be taught regarding warfarin (Coumadin) therapy? **Select all that apply.**
    1. Wear medical identification.
    2. Avoid eating green leafy vegetables.
    3. Keep scheduled blood test appointments.
    4. Use a straight razor when shaving.
    5. Explain the importance of eating green leafy vegetables in a consistent amount.
    6. Review signs and symptoms to report to the health care provider.

12. To prevent thrombophlebitis in the immobilized patient, the nurse should include which of these interventions in the patient's plan of care? **Select all that apply.**
    1. Apply elastic stockings as ordered.
    2. Ambulate as early as the patient's condition allows.
    3. Apply sequential compression devices as ordered.
    4. Delay ambulation with presence of pain upon movement.
    5. Encourage the patient to do leg exercises hourly while in bed.

13. The nurse is planning care for a patient with chronic mitral regurgitation. Which of the following data would be the highest priority for the nurse to collect?
    1. Cardiac rhythm
    2. Heart tones
    3. Peripheral edema
    4. Lung sounds

14. The nurse reviews discharge instructions with the patient who has a history of infective endocarditis. The instructions recommend prophylactic antibiotics when undergoing dental work to prevent which of the following?
    1. Infective endocarditis
    2. Peritonitis
    3. Vegetative emboli
    4. Inflammation

15. A patient, age 46, is admitted for observation with a chest contusion after hitting the steering wheel in a motor vehicle accident. Which of the following findings would be the highest priority?
    1. Bronchovesicular sounds are heard over the major airways.
    2. Chest soreness and tenderness is reported.
    3. Sternal bruising is noted.
    4. Pericardial rub is heard on auscultation.

16. A patient develops postoperative deep vein thrombosis and is started on intravenous heparin. Which of the following laboratory tests does the nurse monitor during heparin therapy?
    1. Plasma fibrinogen
    2. Prothrombin time
    3. Partial thromboplastin time
    4. International normalized ratio

17. The nurse is caring for a patient on warfarin (Coumadin) with an elevated international normalized ratio level. Which of the following would be ordered as the antidote for warfarin?
    1. Vitamin B_{12}
    2. Vitamin K
    3. Calcium chloride
    4. Protamine sulfate

18. Which of the following is a desired outcome for the nursing diagnosis of *Acute Pain* for a patient with acute deep vein thrombosis?
    1. States anxiety is decreased.
    2. States pain is satisfactorily relieved.
    3. Is able to participate in desired activities.
    4. Reports ability to ambulate without pain.

19. A patient visits the doctor for a severe sore throat and fever. As the nurse plans the patient's care, which of the following diagnostic tests is prepared to prevent cardiac complications?
    1. Chest x-ray examination
    2. Throat culture
    3. White blood cell count
    4. Erythrocyte sedimentation rate

20. The nurse is reviewing the daily international normalized ratio for a patient who had a mechanical valve replacement and is prescribed warfarin (Coumadin). The international normalized ratio is 3.7. Which of the following actions should the nurse take now?
    1. Give a dose of warfarin (Coumadin) immediately.
    2. Inform the health care provider.
    3. Give the next scheduled dose of warfarin (Coumadin).
    4. Withhold the next dose of warfarin (Coumadin).

21. A patient who had a hysterectomy 2 days ago reports tenderness in her left calf. Data collection reveals the following: left calf 17.5 inches, right calf 14 inches, left thigh 32 inches, right thigh 28 inches, and a shiny, warm, reddened left leg. Which of the following interventions should be given priority in the patient's plan of care? **Select all that apply.**
    1. Elevate left leg.
    2. Encourage ambulation three times daily.
    3. Encourage bilateral leg exercises.
    4. Apply compression stockings as ordered.
    5. Massage left leg.
    6. Apply warm, moist heat as ordered.

22. Which of the following findings should be reported to the health care provider for a patient receiving warfarin (Coumadin) therapy?
    1. Bleeding time 3 seconds (normal = 2 to 5 seconds)
    2. International normalized ratio 4 (therapeutic = 2 to 3)
    3. Partial thromboplastin time 28 seconds (normal = 30 to 45 seconds)
    4. Prothrombin time 20 seconds (therapeutic = 13.5 to 22 seconds)

23. A patient who has end-stage dilated cardiomyopathy comes to the emergency department with dyspnea. The patient reports waking with a feeling of suffocation, which was frightening. Which of the following responses by the nurse is most appropriate?
    1. "You must have been dreaming."
    2. "Reclining decreases the heart's ability to pump blood."
    3. "Sleeping increases heart rate, which increases the body's need for oxygen."
    4. "Reclining increases fluid returning to the heart, which builds up fluid in the lungs."

24. Which of the following assessments of a patient would indicate a side effect of digoxin (Lanoxin) is occurring that requires follow-up?
    1. Anorexia
    2. Constipation
    3. Hypertension
    4. Skin flushing

25. The health care provider writes a "now" order for codeine 45 mg intramuscular for a patient with thrombophlebitis. The nurse has on hand codeine 60 mg/2 mL. Which of the following doses should be given?
    1. 1.45 mL
    2. 1.5 mL
    3. 1.75 mL
    4. 2.15 mL

26. The nurse checks pedal pulses for a patient who has peripheral arterial disease. Mark the areas where the nurse would palpate pedal pulses.

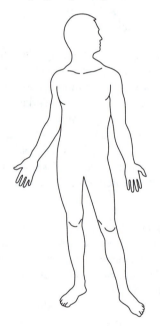

CHAPTER 24
Nursing Care of Patients With Occlusive Cardiovascular Disorders

Name:	
Date:	
Course:	
Instructor:	

AUDIO CASE STUDY

Listen to the audio case study available on Davis Edge and then answer the following questions.

Kathy: Angina and Myocardial Infarction

1. What does the medication nitroglycerin do?

   _____
   _____
   _____

2. How are patients taught to take nitroglycerin?

   _____
   _____
   _____
   _____

3. What symptoms of a heart attack did Mrs. Gallegos have that women may experience without crushing pain?

   _____
   _____
   _____

4. What treatment is ordered for Mrs. Gallegos at the hospital?

_____

_____

_____

VOCABULARY

Match the term with its definition.

1. _____ Lymphangitis
2. _____ Atherosclerosis
3. _____ Stenosis
4. _____ Ischemia
5. _____ Venous stasis ulcer
6. _____ High-density lipoprotein
7. _____ Collateral circulation
8. _____ Balloon angioplasty
9. _____ Angina pectoris
10. _____ Stable angina
11. _____ Unstable angina
12. _____ Varicose veins
13. _____ Raynaud disease
14. _____ Aneurysm
15. _____ Myocardial infarction
16. _____ Troponin I
17. _____ Embolism
18. _____ Thrombus
19. _____ Intermittent claudication
20. _____ Coronary artery disease

1. Tortuous and bulging veins, usually in lower extremity
2. Procedure to compress plaque against wall of artery
3. Chest pain that increases in frequency and is not relieved by rest
4. Inflammation of lymphatic channels
5. Chest pain caused by decreased blood supply to the heart
6. Obstructed blood flow in the coronary arteries
7. Chest pain that usually subsides with rest
8. Venospasms affecting digits with cold exposure
9. Plaque buildup inside arteries
10. Lack of sufficient blood supply
11. A bulging or dilation of an artery
12. Growth of blood vessels to compensate for blocked blood flow
13. Narrowing of a vessel
14. Death of a portion of the myocardium
15. A moving blood clot
16. Protective cholesterol
17. A stationary blood clot
18. Skin breakdown from chronic venous insufficiency
19. Laboratory value that can reflect degree of damage to the heart
20. Exertional calf pain that ceases with rest

ATHEROSCLEROSIS

Answer the following questions.

1. What is the pathophysiology of atherosclerosis?

   _____

   _____

   _____

   _____

   _____

2. What are modifiable risk factors that contribute to atherosclerosis?

   _____

   _____

3. Develop a teaching plan for one of the modifiable risk
   factors for atherosclerosis.

   _____

   _____

   _____

MYOCARDIAL INFARCTION

Find the 26 errors and insert the correct information.

Myocardial infarction (MI) is the death of a portion of the
pericardial sac caused by a blockage or spasm of a coronary
artery. When the patient has an MI, the affected part of the
muscle becomes damaged and no longer functions properly.
Ischemic injury takes several minutes before complete necrosis
and infarction take place. The ischemic process affects the
subendocardial layer, which is the least sensitive to hypoxia.
Myocardial contractility is depressed, so the body attempts
to compensate by triggering the parasympathetic nervous
system. This causes a decrease in myocardial oxygen
demand, which further depresses the myocardium. After

necrosis, the contractility function of the muscle is temporarily
lost. If treatment is initiated after several signs of an MI, the
area of damage can be minimized. If prolonged ischemia
occurs, the size of the infarction can be small.

The area that is affected by an MI depends on which
coronary artery is involved. The left anterior descending
branch of the left main coronary artery is the area that feeds
the lateral wall. The right coronary artery (RCA) feeds the
anterior wall and parts of the atrioventricular node and the
sinoatrial node. An occlusion of the RCA leads to an anterior
MI and to abnormalities of impulse conduction and formation.
The left circumflex coronary artery feeds the inferior wall
and part of the posterior wall of the heart.

Pain is often the least common symptom. The pain does not
radiate. The patient usually believes that an MI is occurring.
Other symptoms may include restlessness; a feeling of
impending doom; nausea; diaphoresis; and hot, clammy, ashen
skin. The only symptom that might be present in the older
adult is vomiting. Men may have atypical symptoms of an MI.

The three strong indicators of an MI are patient history,
abnormal electrocardiographic readings, and high triglyceride
levels.

Initially, patients are kept on bedrest to increase myocardial
oxygen demand. Patients are medicated promptly when

experiencing chest pain. Codeine is the most widely used narcotic for MI. It helps decrease anxiety, slows respirations, and vasoconstricts the coronary arteries. Oxygen is given usually at 1 L/min via nasal cannula. Nitroglycerin orally, topical, or by intravenous (IV) drip can also be administered. Percutaneous coronary intervention is a frequent treatment option for an occluded coronary vein.

A nursing care plan should include factors that may contribute to decreased cardiac workload. Patient and family teaching topics include diet, stress reduction, exercise, smoking cessation, and medications.

PHARMACOLOGICAL TREATMENT

Match the medication to the appropriate description.

1. _____ Eptifibatide (Integrilin)
2. _____ Metoprolol (Lopressor)
3. _____ Nitroglycerin
4. _____ Heparin
5. _____ Cholestyramine (Questran)
6. _____ Clopidogrel (Plavix)
7. _____ Atorvastatin (Lipitor)
8. _____ Reteplase (Retavase)
9. _____ Amlodipine (Norvasc)
10. _____ Isosorbide dinitrate (Isordil)

1. Drug of choice for anginal attacks
2. Bile acid sequestrant
3. Beta blocker
4. Calcium channel blocker
5. Thrombolytic
6. Antiplatelet
7. Does not dissolve existing clots
8. Glycoprotein IIb/IIIa inhibitor
9. Long-acting nitrate
10. Reduces cholesterol synthesis

CRITICAL THINKING

Read the following case study and answer the questions.

Mr. Edwards is a 43-year-old man with a history of peripheral vascular disease and hypertension. He smokes two packs of cigarettes per day. He reports calf pain during minimal exercise that decreases with rest.

1. Circle the **priority** nursing diagnosis related to Mr. Edwards's symptoms, and write a patient outcome for it.
   1. *Ineffective Peripheral Tissue Perfusion* related to compromised circulation
   2. *Fatigue* related to pain on exertion
   3. *Impaired Physical Mobility* related to pain and muscle spasms
   4. *Ineffective Coping* related to stress associated with pain

   _____

   _____

   _____

2. Explain what happens when intermittent claudication occurs. _____

   _____

   _____

   _____

3. Why does rest decrease the pain? _____

   _____

   _____

4. Describe how smoking contributes to decreased circulation. _____

   _____

   _____

   _____

   _____

REVIEW QUESTIONS—CONTENT REVIEW

Choose the best answer unless directed otherwise.

1. The nurse is assisting with a community teaching session on atherosclerosis. Place in order the multistep process in the development of atherosclerosis that the nurse would explain to attendees.
   1. Injury occurs to the endothelial cells that line the walls of the arteries
   2. Lipids, platelets, and other clotting factors accumulate
   3. Inflammation results
   4. The growth of smooth muscle cells is stimulated
   5. Plaque builds up
   6. Scar tissue replaces some of the arterial wall

2. A patient hospitalized with a myocardial infarction suddenly begins having severe respiratory distress with frothy sputum. These signs indicate that the patient is developing which of the following complications?
   1. Cardiac tamponade
   2. Pneumonia
   3. Pneumothorax
   4. Pulmonary edema

3. As the nurse gathers data on a patient's circulation in the lower extremities, which of the following findings would indicate decreased arterial circulation? **Select all that apply.**
   1. Absent leg hair
   2. Capillary refill less than 3 seconds
   3. Diminished pulses
   4. Thickened toenails
   5. Stasis ulcer

4. The nurse is teaching the patient about controlling cholesterol with diet. Which of the following dietary actions may reduce cholesterol? **Select all that apply.**
   1. Avoiding trans fats
   2. Consuming whole grains
   3. Limiting fruit intake
   4. Drinking whole milk
   5. Reducing saturated fats
   6. Limiting sugar-sweetened beverages

5. The nurse understands that pain associated with coronary artery disease occurs from which of the following?
   1. Lack of nutrients to the heart
   2. Interrupted electrical activity to areas of the heart
   3. Lack of sufficient oxygen to the myocardium
   4. Increased cardiac workload

REVIEW QUESTIONS—TEST PREPARATION

Choose the best answer unless directed otherwise.

6. A patient who has been scheduled for an exercise stress electrocardiogram asks why this test is needed. Which of the following is the nurse's best response?
   1. "It can predict whether a heart attack may occur."
   2. "It identifies how much more exercise is needed."
   3. "It determines a target heart rate."
   4. "It shows how the heart performs during exercise."

7. During an exercise stress electrocardiogram, a patient reports chest pain, and the test is stopped. When the patient is asked to undergo a heart catheterization, the patient appears apprehensive and worried. Which of the following is the most appropriate action for the nurse to take to reduce the patient's anxiety?
   1. Explain how coronary artery disease is treated.
   2. Avoid discussing the heart catheterization to help the patient relax.
   3. Explain how well others have done after having this procedure.
   4. Listen to the patient express feelings about the situation.

8. Which of the following statements by a patient demonstrates to the nurse that the patient understands when to replace prescribed nitroglycerin tablets?
   1. "Pills no longer cause tingling sensation when used."
   2. "Pills disintegrate when touched."
   3. "Pills smell like vinegar."
   4. "Pills become discolored."

9. After hospitalization for a myocardial infarction, a patient is placed on a low-sodium diet. In discussing foods allowed on this diet, the nurse should inform the patient that this includes which of the following?
   1. Hot dogs
   2. Fresh vegetables
   3. Milk and cheese
   4. Canned soups

10. Which of the following does the nurse correctly include in a teaching plan as modifiable risk factors for coronary artery disease? **Select all that apply.**
    1. Hypertension
    2. Gender
    3. Age
    4. Smoking
    5. Diabetes mellitus

11. Which of the following should the nurse correctly include in a teaching plan as being high in saturated fat? **Select all that apply.**
    1. Avocado
    2. Tuna fish
    3. Beef
    4. Olive oil
    5. Cheddar cheese
    6. Coconut oil

12. The nurse is collecting data on a patient. Which of the following clinical manifestations would the nurse expect to find with acute venous insufficiency? **Select all that apply.**
    1. Full superficial veins
    2. An aching, cramping type of pain
    3. Absence of edema
    4. Cool and cyanotic skin
    5. Hyperemia

13. The nurse understands that which of the following are the most characteristic symptoms of Buerger disease? **Select all that apply.**
    1. Numbness
    2. Pain
    3. Cramping
    4. Swelling
    5. Bounding pulses
    6. Intermittent claudication

14. A patient has been diagnosed with Raynaud disease and asks the nurse what occurs with this disease. Which of the following is the most appropriate response?
    1. "Arterial vessel occlusion is caused by many clots that develop in the heart and are carried to the bloodstream."
    2. "Arteriolar vasoconstriction occurs, most often in the fingertips with symptoms of coldness, pain, and pale skin."
    3. "Peripheral vasospasm occurs in the lower limbs as a result of valve damage from long-standing venous stasis."
    4. "Thrombosis related to prolonged vasoconstriction caused by overexposure to the cold occurs."

15. The nurse is providing teaching to a patient with Buerger disease. Which of the following statements by the patient would the nurse evaluate as indicating understanding about Buerger disease?
    1. "Smoking cessation is important because nicotine is a vasoconstrictor."
    2. "Those most affected are middle-aged women after menopause."
    3. "A low-fat diet is required to reduce atherosclerosis in large arteries."
    4. "Adequate fluid intake is important to maintain blood pressure."

16. Mark two common insertion sites for the catheter during a cardiac catheterization that the nurse would monitor postprocedure.

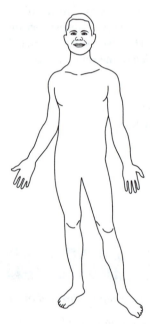

CHAPTER 25
Nursing Care of Patients With Cardiac Arrhythmias

Name:	
Date:	
Course:	
Instructor:	

AUDIO CASE STUDY

Listen to the audio case study available on Davis Edge and then answer the following questions.

Sandy and Identification and Care of Dysrhythmias

1. What are the six steps for dysrhythmia (also called arrhythmia) interpretation?

_____

_____

_____

_____

2. What might missing P waves indicate?

_____

_____

_____

_____

3. What are normal PR interval and QRS interval measurements?

_____

_____

_____

_____

4. What type of initial pacemaker did Mr. Ragland require for third-degree heart block?

_____

_____

_____

VOCABULARY

Match the words and definitions.

1. _____ Amplitude
2. _____ Atrial depolarization
3. _____ Atrial systole
4. _____ Bigeminy
5. _____ Cardioversion
6. _____ Complete heart block
7. _____ Contractility
8. _____ Decompensation
9. _____ Defibrillate
10. _____ Inherent
11. _____ Ischemia
12. _____ Isoelectric line
13. _____ Multifocal
14. _____ Unifocal
15. _____ Right bundle branch block
16. _____ Trigeminy
17. _____ Quadrigeminy
18. _____ Ventricular diastole
19. _____ Ventricular escape rhythm
20. _____ Ventricular repolarization
21. _____ Ventricular systole

1. Beat occurring every fourth complex, as in premature ventricular contractions (PVCs)
2. Belonging to anything naturally
3. Coming or originating from one site
4. Condition in which there is a complete dissociation between atrial and ventricular systoles
5. Contraction of the atria
6. Contraction of the two ventricles
7. Disturbance in heart conduction system in which right bundle is blocked and does not conduct impulses normally
8. Elective procedure in which synchronized shock of 25 to 50 joules is delivered to restore normal sinus rhythm
9. Electrical activation of the atria
10. Electrical tracing is neither positive nor negative; baseline
11. Failure of the heart to maintain adequate circulation
12. Force with which left ventricular ejection occurs
13. Local deficiency of blood supply resulting from obstruction of the circulation to the area
14. Occurring every third beat, as in PVCs
15. Occurring every second beat, as in PVCs
16. Originating from many foci or sites
17. Period of relaxation of the ventricle
18. Reestablishment of the polarized state of the muscle after contraction
19. Size, height, or fullness of voltage
20. Naturally occurring rhythm of the ventricles when the rest of the conduction system fails
21. Use of electrical device to apply countershocks to the heart through electrodes placed on the chest wall

COMPONENTS OF A CARDIAC CYCLE

Label the components of a cardiac cycle.

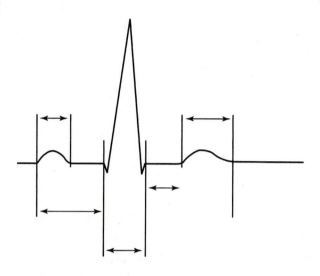

HEART RATE

Calculate the heart rate using the 6-second method.

1.

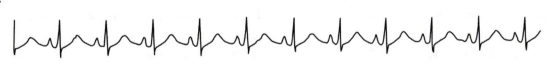

Heart rate = _____

2.

Heart rate = _____

3.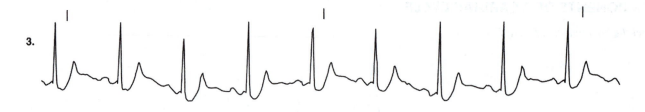

Heart rate = _____

CARDIAC CONDUCTION

Match the words and definitions.

1. _____ Sinoatrial node
2. _____ Atrioventricular node
3. _____ Normal sinus rhythm
4. _____ Right atrium
5. _____ Right ventricle
6. _____ Left atrium
7. _____ Left ventricle
8. _____ Bradycardia
9. _____ Tachycardia
10. _____ Q wave
11. _____ P wave
12. _____ R wave
13. _____ S wave
14. _____ T wave
15. _____ U wave
16. _____ Premature
17. _____ Sinus tachycardia
18. _____ Sinus bradycardia
19. _____ Premature atrial contraction
20. _____ Atrial fibrillation
21. _____ Premature ventricular contraction
22. _____ Ventricular tachycardia
23. _____ Ventricular fibrillation
24. _____ Asystole

1. Heart rate less than 60
2. Flat line with no QRS complexes seen on ECG
3. An early beat
4. An early beat that has a P wave and a normal QRS complex
5. Where normal cardiac impulse originates
6. A chaotic pattern; no visible cardiac cycles
7. No identifiable P waves with a normal QRS complex; irregularly irregular rhythm
8. Wave that precedes a QRS complex
9. Where an impulse is delayed before going to the Purkinje fibers
10. An early beat with no P wave and a wide, bizarre QRS complex
11. Successive beats of three or more wide, bizarre QRS complexes
12. Rhythm with normal P waves, QRS complex, and T waves with a heart rate of 60 to 100 beats per minute (bpm)
13. The first negative deflection of a QRS complex
14. A small wave rarely seen after the T wave
15. The first positive deflection of a QRS complex
16. Rhythm with normal P waves, QRS complex, and T waves with a heart rate of less than 60 bpm
17. The chamber of the heart that pumps the blood to the rest of the body
18. The chamber that receives blood from the body.
19. Rhythm with normal P waves, QRS complex, and T waves with a heart rate of more than 100 bpm
20. The wave that follows the QRS complex
21. The chamber that receives blood from the pulmonary veins
22. The downward deflection after the R wave
23. Heart rate of more than 100 bpm
24. Chamber that propels blood into the pulmonary artery

ELECTROCARDIOGRAM INTERPRETATION

Analyze the electrocardiogram (ECG) rhythms using the six-step interpretation process.

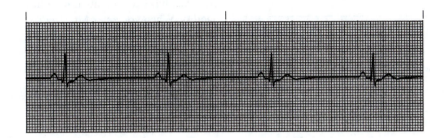

A.

1. Rhythm: _____

2. Heart rate: _____

3. P waves: _____

4. PR interval: _____

5. QRS interval: _____

6. QT interval: _____

7. ECG interpretation: _____

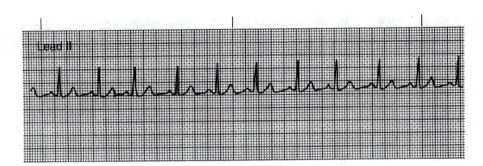

B.

1. Rhythm: _____

2. Heart rate: _____

3. P waves: _____

4. PR interval: _____

5. QRS interval: _____

6. QT interval: _____

7. ECG interpretation: _____

CRITICAL THINKING: MRS. SAMUELS

Read the following case study and answer the questions.

Mrs. Samuels is admitted to the hospital for chest pain. Tests are done. Her ECG shows bigeminal PVCs of more than 6 per minute that are close to the T wave. Her potassium level is 2.8 mEq/L. She is short of breath on exertion. Her blood pressure is 104/56 mm Hg, pulse is 72 bpm, and respirations are 16 breaths per minute.

1. What should you do first? _____
   _____
   _____
   _____

2. What actions should you take regarding the arrhythmia?

_____

_____

_____

_____

3. What are some causes for this arrhythmia? _____

_____

_____

4. What additional symptoms might you anticipate?

_____

_____

_____

5. What type of orders should you expect from the health care provider? _____

_____

_____

_____

CRITICAL THINKING: MR. PEET

Read the following case study and answer the questions.

Mr. Peet has been admitted to your unit in a long-term care facility. When you enter Mr. Peet's room, you note that he is having difficulty breathing and is unresponsive.

1. What are your initial actions?

_____

_____

2. What should you do after finding no pulse or respirations? _____

_____

3. What is your responsibility during a cardiac/respiratory arrest code? _____

_____

REVIEW QUESTIONS—CONTENT REVIEW

Choose the best answer unless directed otherwise.

1. The nurse understands that which of the following is represented by a cardiac cycle on an electrocardiogram?
   1. Circulation of the blood through the body
   2. Circulation of the blood through the heart
   3. Depolarization and repolarization of the four heart chambers
   4. Pumping action of the heart

2. The heart receives blood returning from the body through which of the following?
   1. Pulmonary vein
   2. Aorta
   3. Vena cavae
   4. Right coronary artery

3. Which of the following separates the right side of the heart from the left?
   1. Chamber
   2. Pericardium
   3. Valve
   4. Septum

4. Which of the following chambers of the heart has the thickest myocardium and greatest workload?
   1. Left ventricle
   2. Right ventricle
   3. Right atrium
   4. Left atrium

5. Which of the following waveforms represents the resting state of the ventricle on the electrocardiogram?
   1. P wave
   2. QRS complex
   3. U wave
   4. T wave

6. Which of the following is the normal rate for the sinoatrial node?
   1. 20 to 40 beats per minute
   2. 40 to 60 beats per minute
   3. 60 to 100 beats per minute
   4. More than 100 beats per minute

7. The nurse understands that rhythms arising from the primary pacing node of the heart are referred to as which of the following?
   1. Escape beats
   2. Bundle branch blocks
   3. Sinus rhythms
   4. Ectopic rhythms

REVIEW QUESTIONS—TEST PREPARATION

Choose the best answer unless directed otherwise.

8. The nurse sees a life-threatening arrhythmia on a patient's cardiac monitor. Which of the following actions should the nurse take first?
   1. Notify the health care provider immediately.
   2. Examine the patient.
   3. Administer antiarrhythmic medication.
   4. Obtain vital signs.

9. The nurse is teaching a patient about digoxin (Lanoxin). The nurse would evaluate the patient as understanding the teaching if the patient made which of these statements? **Select all that apply.**
   1. "Digoxin decreases ectopic beats."
   2. "The force of heart contractions is increased with digoxin."
   3. "The resting heart rate increases when digoxin is taken."
   4. "Digoxin raises blood pressure."
   5. "Digoxin slows the heart rate."

10. The nurse is providing care to a patient with atrial fibrillation. Which of the following statements, if made by the patient, would be of the most concern?
    1. "Warfarin required frequent lab testing, so I quit taking it."
    2. "It seems like my feet are a little swollen."
    3. "My wife and I got a membership at the local health club."
    4. "I've been having trouble falling asleep at night."

11. The nurse is collecting data on a patient who has been treated for atrial fibrillation. Which prescribed treatments would the nurse anticipate could be reported by the patient for treatment of the atrial fibrillation? **Select all that apply.**
    1. Amiodarone
    2. Nitroglycerin
    3. Warfarin (Coumadin)
    4. Digoxin (Lanoxin)
    5. Synchronized cardioversion
    6. Epinephrine

12. The nurse is caring for a patient who has had three or more premature ventricular contractions occurring in a row on the electrocardiogram tracing. The nurse should document this as which of the following?
    1. Ventricular tachycardia
    2. Bigeminy
    3. Trigeminy
    4. Multifocal premature ventricular contractions

13. The nurse is caring for a patient experiencing ventricular tachycardia who is stable. Which of the following would the nurse recognize as being the initial treatment for this arrhythmia?
    1. Cardioversion
    2. Pacemaker
    3. Defibrillation
    4. Intravenous antiarrhythmic medication

14. The nurse is caring for a patient whose cardiac monitor shows a total absence of electrical impulse with a flat line. The nurse does not detect a pulse or blood pressure. The nurse would document this as which of the following rhythms?
    1. Asystole
    2. Atrial flutter
    3. Atrial fibrillation
    4. Ventricular fibrillation

15. A patient with a cardiac disorder is having increased premature ventricular contractions and feels "anxious." After vital signs are obtained, what actions should the nurse take? **Select all that apply.**
    1. Order an electrocardiogram and cardiac enzymes.
    2. Call the health care provider.
    3. Elevate the head of the bed.
    4. Allow the patient to rest alone.
    5. Start oxygen at 2 L/min
    6. Place bed in modified Trendelenburg position.

16. The nurse is caring for a patient who is fatigued and undergoing cardiac testing. For which of the following arrhythmias would the nurse anticipate the patient's need for a permanent pacemaker? **Select all that apply.**
    1. Ventricular fibrillation
    2. First-degree atrioventricular block
    3. Atrial fibrillation
    4. Third-degree atrioventricular block
    5. Symptomatic bradycardia
    6. Premature atrial contractions

17. A patient who is on a cardiac monitor reports feeling an irregular heartbeat to the nurse. The nurse observes premature ventricular contractions on the cardiac monitor and prints an electrocardiogram strip. Mark the premature ventricular contractions seen on the strip.

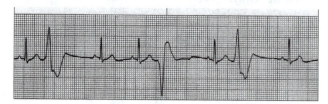

18. The nurse is observing the electrocardiogram strip of a patient with a dual-chamber pacemaker for proper functioning. Mark the ventricular pacemaker spikes on the strip.

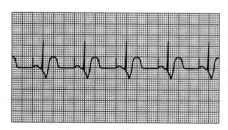

19. The nurse is present at a school event when a person states the presence of chest pain and collapses. The nurse obtains the automatic external defibrillator to place on the person. Mark the two areas on the person where the nurse should attach the automatic external defibrillator pads.

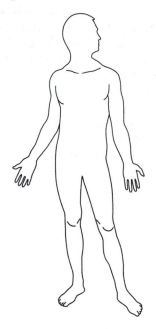

20. The nurse is viewing the patient's permanent pacemaker incision for signs of infection. Mark the two areas where the nurse would look to locate the subcutaneous incision for the pacemaker.

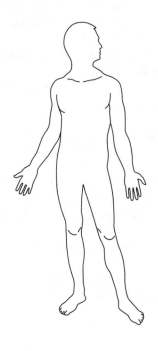

CHAPTER 26
Nursing Care of Patients With Heart Failure

Name:	_____
Date:	_____
Course:	_____
Instructor:	_____

AUDIO CASE STUDY

Listen to the audio case study available on Davis Edge and then answer the following questions.

Mrs. Sims and Heart Failure

1. What signs and symptoms of right- and left-sided heart failure (HF) did Mrs. Sims have?

_____
_____
_____
_____

2. What treatment for HF was provided for Mrs. Sims?

_____
_____

3. What acute complication did Mrs. Sims develop in the hospital?

_____
_____

4. What treatment was Mrs. Sims given for this complication?

_____
_____
_____
_____

VOCABULARY

Fill in the blank with the appropriate term found in the word list.

Afterload   Peripheral vascular resistance

Cor pulmonale   Preload

Hepatomegaly   Pulmonary Edema

Orthopnea   Splenomegaly

Paroxysmal nocturnal dyspnea

1. _____ is the acute inability of the heart to pump enough blood to meet the
   body's oxygen and nutrient needs.

2. _____ occurs when the right side of the heart fails because of an increased
   workload caused by pulmonary disease.

3. Organ enlargement that may occur with right-sided HF is known as _____
   and _____.

4. The goal of treatment for HF is to improve the heart's pumping ability and decrease the heart's workload
   by reducing _____.

5. _____ causes supine patients to awaken suddenly with a feeling of suffocation.

6. The end-diastole stretch in the ventricles produced by ventricular volume is _____.

7. The tension in the ventricular wall during systole necessary to overcome vascular resistance
   is _____.

8. _____ is dyspnea that occurs when the patient lies down.

FLUID ACCUMULATION PATTERNS

Label the backward accumulation of fluid and shade areas of fluid congestion.

The heart pumps blood in a closed circuit. If one side of the heart fails to adequately pump blood forward, it pools and backs up from the failing chamber. On the drawing, use arrows to mark the path of the backward accumulation of fluid from the side of the heart that is failing. Shade in areas where fluid congestion occurs.

To increase your understanding of where the backward accumulation of fluid occurs from a certain side of the heart, use blue shading to illustrate the side with deoxygenated blood accumulation. Use red shading for the side with oxygenated blood accumulation.

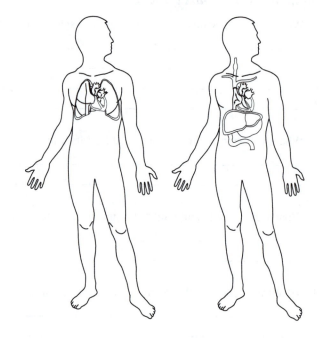

SIGNS AND SYMPTOMS OF HEART FAILURE

In HF, certain signs and symptoms occur based on the side of the heart that is failing as a pump.

Match the following sign or symptom to the failing side of the heart that is causing it.

1. _____ Dry cough
2. _____ Peripheral edema
3. _____ Crackles
4. _____ Hepatomegaly
5. _____ Jugular vein distention
6. _____ Dyspnea
7. _____ Splenomegaly
8. _____ Orthopnea

1. Left-sided HF
2. Right-sided HF

CRITICAL THINKING

Read the following case study and answer the questions.

Mr. Donner, age 72, is admitted to the cardiac unit for increasing dyspnea on exertion and fatigue.

Subjective Data

• History of HF for 2 years
• Unable to walk one block without increasing dyspnea
• Sleeps at 60-degree angle in reclining chair
• Increasing fatigue during the last 2 weeks

Objective Data

• Blood pressure 140/78 mm Hg, pulse 108 beats per minute, respirations 24 breaths per minute, temperature 98.8°F (37.1°C)
• Jugular vein distention at 45 degrees
• Has frequent dry cough
• Bilateral crackles in lung bases
• Nonpitting edema
• Chest x-ray examination: left and right ventricular hypertrophy, bilateral fluid in lower lung lobes

1. Explain the cause of Mr. Donner's fatigue, cough, and shortness of breath. _____
   _____
   _____

2. Which of Mr. Donner's signs and symptoms are from left-sided HF and which are from right-sided HF?
   Left: _____
   Right: _____

3. Explain the purpose of each of the following therapies. How would they be beneficial in treating Mr. Donner's heart failure?
   1. Furosemide (Lasix) 40 mg by mouth twice daily: _____
      _____
      _____

   2. Lisinopril (Zestril) 5 mg by mouth daily: _____
      _____

   3. 2-g sodium diet: _____
      _____

   4. Oxygen 4 L/min: _____
      _____
      _____

4. Mr. Donner suddenly becomes dyspneic and anxious. He has moist crackles throughout his lungs and pink frothy sputum. Explain what is happening. _____
   _____
   _____
   _____

5. Explain the purpose of each of the following therapies. How are they beneficial in treating Mr. Donner's acute HF?
   1. High Fowler position: _____
      _____
      _____
      _____

   2. Oxygen 6 L/min: _____
      _____
      _____
      _____

   3. Furosemide (Lasix) intravenous push (IVP): _____
      _____
      _____
      _____

   4. Nitroglycerin IV infusion: _____
      _____
      _____
      _____

6. List two priority nursing diagnoses and goals for Mr. Donner's chronic HF.

_____

_____

_____

_____

_____

7. What are Mr. Donner's health learning needs to manage his chronic condition?

_____

_____

_____

_____

_____

_____

REVIEW QUESTIONS—CONTENT REVIEW

Choose the best answer unless directed otherwise.

1. A patient is being given digoxin (Lanoxin) to treat heart failure. Which of the following are within the usual adult daily dosage range for digoxin (Lanoxin)? **Select all that apply.**
   1. 0.005 mg
   2. 0.025 mg
   3. 0.125 mg
   4. 0.25 mg
   5. 0.5 mg
   6. 2.5 mg

2. When the nurse is reviewing a patient's daily laboratory test results, which of the following electrolyte imbalances should the nurse recognize as predisposing the patient to digoxin (Lanoxin) toxicity?
   1. Hypokalemia
   2. Hyperkalemia
   3. Hyponatremia
   4. Hypernatremia

3. If a patient has elevated pulmonary vascular pressures, the nurse understands that the patient is most likely to develop which of the following physiological cardiac changes?
   1. Left atrial atrophy
   2. Right atrial atrophy
   3. Left ventricular hypertrophy
   4. Right ventricular hypertrophy

REVIEW QUESTIONS—TEST PREPARATION

Choose the best answer unless directed otherwise.

4. A patient is admitted to a medical unit with a diagnosis of heart failure. The patient reports increasing fatigue during the past 2 weeks. Which of the following is the most likely cause of this fatigue?
   1. Dyspnea
   2. Decreased cardiac output
   3. Dry cough
   4. Orthopnea

5. A patient asks the nurse what a diagnosis of heart failure means. Which of the following is the nurse's best response?
   1. "Your heart briefly stops."
   2. "Your heart has an area of muscle that is dead."
   3. "Your heart is pumping too much blood."
   4. "Your heart is not an efficient pump."

6. A patient's chest x-ray examination indicates fluid in both lung bases. Which of the following signs or symptoms present during the nurse's data collection most reflects these x-ray examination findings?
   1. Fatigue
   2. Peripheral edema
   3. Bilateral crackles
   4. Jugular vein distention

7. To monitor the severity of a patient's heart failure, which of the following information is the most appropriate for the nurse to gather daily?
   1. Weight
   2. Calorie count
   3. Appetite
   4. Abdominal girth

8. Which of the following signs indicates to the nurse that digoxin (Lanoxin) has been effective for a patient?
   1. Urine output decreases
   2. Urine output increases
   3. Heart rate higher than 95 beats per minute
   4. Heart rate lower than 50 beats per minute

9. For a patient who is being discharged on digoxin (Lanoxin), the nurse should include which of the following in an explanation on the signs and symptoms of digoxin toxicity? **Select all that apply.**
   1. Poor appetite
   2. Constipation
   3. Halos around lights
   4. Apnea
   5. Yellow lights
   6. Bradycardia

10. The patient is being discharged on furosemide (Lasix). The nurse evaluates the patient as understanding medication teaching if the patient states that which of the following laboratory tests will be monitored as ordered?
    1. "I will have my urine sodium checked."
    2. "I will have my calcium level checked."
    3. "I will have my prothrombin time checked."
    4. "I will have my potassium level checked."

11. The nurse would evaluate the patient as understanding management of chronic heart failure if the patient stated which of the following? **Select all that apply.**
    1. "I will weigh myself at the same time each day."
    2. "I will cook with salt."
    3. "I will report the occurrence of edema."
    4. "I will take my diuretic as needed for edema."
    5. "I will eat fresh vegetables."

12. The nurse evaluates that bumetanide (Bumex) given intravenously is effective in treating pulmonary edema if which of the following patient signs or symptoms is resolved?
    1. Pedal edema
    2. Jugular venous distention
    3. Pink, frothy sputum
    4. Bradycardia

13. A patient is being taught the action of digoxin (Lanoxin), which is an inotropic agent. The nurse defines an inotropic agent as a medication that has which of the following actions?
    1. Decreases heart rate
    2. Increases heart rate
    3. Increases conduction time
    4. Strengthens heart contraction

14. For a patient receiving furosemide (Lasix), the nurse evaluates the medication as being effective if which of the following effects occurs?
    1. Bilateral crackles diminish.
    2. Serum potassium decreases.
    3. Heart rate increases.
    4. Pulse pressure increases.

15. When caring for an anxious patient with dyspnea, which of the following nursing actions is most helpful to include in the plan of care to relieve anxiety?
    1. Increase activity levels.
    2. Stay at patient's bedside.
    3. Pull the privacy curtain.
    4. Close the patient's door.

16. Mark the area where congestion occurs from left-sided heart failure.

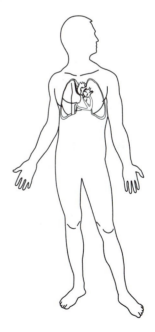

17. Mark the area where the nurse would monitor for peripheral edema that occurs from right-sided heart failure.

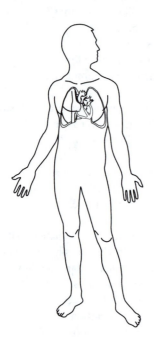

18. Mark the area where the nurse would auscultate for congestion occurring in acute heart failure.

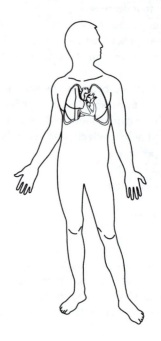

CHAPTER 27

Hematologic and Lymphatic System Function, Assessment, and Therapeutic Measures

Name: _____

Date: _____

Course: _____

Instructor: _____

AUDIO CASE STUDY

Listen to the audio case study available on Davis Edge and then answer the following questions.

Mrs. Casey Receives Blood

1. How long did Jodi stay in the room after the blood reached Mrs. Casey's vein?

   _____

   _____

2. What kind of reaction did Mrs. Casey have?

   _____

   _____

3. What treatment was ordered?

   _____

   _____

4. How long can a blood transfusion safely hang?

   _____

   _____

VOCABULARY

Fill in the blank with the appropriate word.

1. _____ is a large hemorrhage under the skin.

2. _____ is the term used to describe swelling from blockage of lymph circulation.

3. Tiny hemorrhages into the skin creating a polka-dot appearance are called _____.

4. _____ is caused by hemorrhages into the skin, mucous membranes, or internal organs.

5. The patient with _____ has an increased risk for bleeding because of insufficient platelets.

LYMPHATIC SYSTEM REVIEW

Match each part of the lymphatic system with its proper description.

1. _____ Lymph capillaries

2. _____ Lymph nodules

3. _____ Thoracic duct

4. _____ Lymph nodes

5. _____ Valves

1. Destroy pathogens in the lymph from the extremities before the lymph is returned to the blood

2. Collect tissue fluid from intercellular spaces

3. Prevent backflow of lymph in larger lymph vessels

4. Destroy pathogens that penetrate mucous membranes

5. Empties lymph from the lower body and upper left quadrant into the left subclavian vein

STRUCTURES OF THE LYMPHATIC SYSTEM

Label the following structures.

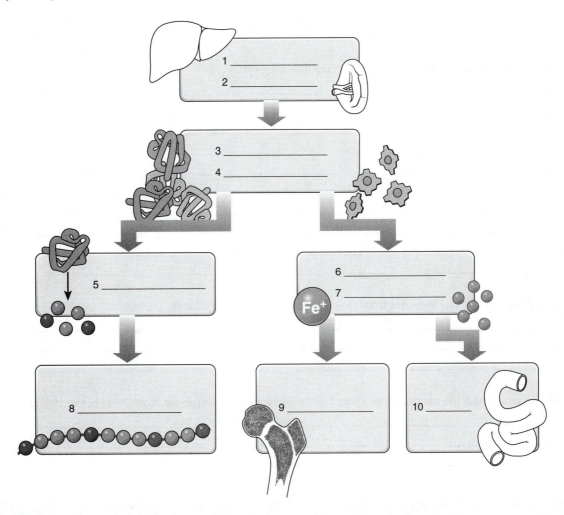

HEMATOLOGIC SYSTEM REVIEW

Match each term with its definition.

1. _____ Albumin
2. _____ Macrophages
3. _____ Calcium ions
4. _____ Intrinsic factor
5. _____ Hemoglobin
6. _____ Basophils
7. _____ Red bone marrow
8. _____ Stem cell
9. _____ Megakaryocyte
10. _____ Lymphocytes

1. May become any kind of blood cell
2. Essential for chemical clotting
3. Release histamine
4. A hematopoietic tissue
5. May become cells that produce antibodies
6. Large phagocytic cells
7. Promotes absorption of vitamin B_{12}
8. Its fragments become platelets
9. Carries oxygen in red blood cells
10. Pulls tissue fluid into capillaries to maintain blood volume

CRITICAL THINKING

Read the case study and answer the questions.

Mr. Foster is receiving a unit of packed red blood cells. You assist with identification of the patient before the transfusion begins. The registered nurse then delegates monitoring of his vital signs every half hour to you.

1. Why should Mr. Foster be monitored for each of the following symptoms?

Fever _____

_____

Back pain _____

_____

Respiratory distress _____

_____

Crackles _____

_____

Hives _____

_____

2. Mr. Foster's respiratory rate increases from 16 to 20 breaths per minute. What do you do?

_____

_____

_____

3. The physician asks that the transfusion be slowed down. How many hours can the blood hang before it must be stopped?

_____

_____

_____

REVIEW QUESTIONS—CONTENT REVIEW

Choose the best answer unless directed otherwise.

1. What is the mineral necessary for chemical clotting?
   1. Iron
   2. Sodium
   3. Potassium
   4. Calcium

2. Through which of the following does lymph return to the blood?
   1. Carotid arteries
   2. Aorta
   3. Inferior vena cava
   4. Subclavian veins

3. Which of the following is a normal hemoglobin value?
   1. 38% to 48%
   2. 12 to 18 g/100 mL
   3. 48 to 54 mg %
   4. 27 to 36 g/dL

4. Which laboratory study is monitored for the patient receiving heparin therapy?
   1. International normalized ratio
   2. Prothrombin time
   3. Partial thromboplastin time
   4. Bleeding time

5. Which blood product replaces missing clotting factors in the patient who has a bleeding disorder?
   1. Platelets
   2. Packed red blood cells
   3. Albumin
   4. Cryoprecipitate

6. Which of the following items are transported in blood plasma? **Select all that apply.**
   1. Oxygen
   2. Nutrients
   3. Carbon dioxide
   4. Hormones
   5. Wastes
   6. Electrolytes

REVIEW QUESTIONS—TEST PREPARATION

Choose the best answer unless directed otherwise.

7. A patient is on warfarin (Coumadin) therapy and has an international normalized ratio of 1.6. Which action by the nurse is appropriate?
   1. Observe the patient for abnormal bleeding.
   2. Notify the physician and expect an order to increase the warfarin dose.
   3. Advise the patient to double today's dose of warfarin.
   4. Administer vitamin K per protocol.

8. A patient receiving a transfusion of packed red blood cells reports chest and back pain. How should the nurse respond?
   1. Do a complete head-to-toe examination.
   2. Ask the patient to rate the pain on a 0 to 10 scale.
   3. Stop the transfusion and call the registered nurse immediately depending on agency policy.
   4. Administer an analgesic, as needed.

9. The nurse is preparing to assist the physician with a bone marrow biopsy. Which of the following interventions is most important for the nurse to carry out before the procedure?
   1. Explain the procedure to the patient's family.
   2. Administer an analgesic to the patient.
   3. Observe the patient for bleeding.
   4. Drape the biopsy site.

10. The nurse is providing care for patients on a medical surgical unit. Which of the following patients is at increased risk for infection?
    1. A 57-year-old with a white blood cell count of 6,500/mm^3
    2. A 63-year-old with a platelet count of 110,000/mm^3
    3. A 49-year-old with a hematocrit level of 44%
    4. An 88-year-old with a neutrophil count of 32%

11. The nurse is providing care for a patient who is admitted to the hospital with left inguinal swelling. Mark the area the nurse should assess for swelling.

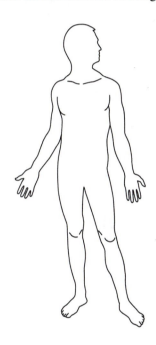

CHAPTER 28
Nursing Care of Patients With Hematologic and Lymphatic Disorders

Name:	_____
Date:	_____
Course:	_____
Instructor:	_____

AUDIO CASE STUDY

Listen to the audio case study available on Davis Edge and then answer the following questions.

Lloyd and Chronic Myelogenous Leukemia

1. How did Lloyd first learn he had leukemia?

   _____
   _____
   _____
   _____

2. What nursing care is important prior to assisting with a patient having a bone marrow biopsy?

   _____
   _____
   _____
   _____

3. Why does Lloyd need to be careful with gardening?

   _____
   _____
   _____
   _____

VOCABULARY

Label each statement true or false and correct false statements.

1. _____ Anemia is a reduction in white blood cells.

2. _____ Hemolysis is the destruction of red blood cells.

3. _____ Pancytopenia is reduced numbers of all blood cells.

4. _____ Polycythemia is the production of excess blood cells.

5. _____ Phlebotomy is the excision of a vessel.

6. _____ Disseminated intravascular coagulation involves accelerated clotting throughout the circulation.

7. _____ Thrombocytopenia is an increase in platelets.

8. _____ Hemarthrosis is bleeding into the muscles.

9. _____ Leukemia literally means "white blood."

10. _____ Cancer of the lymph system is called *lymphemia*.

11. _____ Abnormalities in B cells and T cells can result in lymphoma.

12. _____ Enlargement of the spleen is called *splenomegaly*.

CRITICAL THINKING: LEUKEMIA

Read the case study and answer the questions.

Mr. Frantzis is a 60-year-old man in the acute stage of chronic lymphocytic leukemia. He is admitted to a nursing home because he has no family to help care for him. He has had chemotherapy in the past but has decided against further treatment. You are assigned to his care today. You find him pale and weak, with no energy to get out of bed. He also reports pain in his chest.

1. Mr. Frantzis says he is too weak to get up for breakfast. What should you do? _____

_____

_____

_____

2. How do you follow up on the pain in his chest? _____

_____

_____

_____

3. The nursing assistant assigned to Mr. Frantzis has a runny nose. What should you do? _____

_____

_____

_____

4. Mr. Frantzis calls you "Jennifer" when you enter his room, but that is not your name. How do you respond?

_____

_____

_____

_____

_____

5. You note bleeding from Mr. Frantzis's gums. What care can you provide? _____

_____

_____

_____

CRITICAL THINKING: HODGKIN DISEASE

Circle the five errors in the following paragraph and write in the correct information.

Joe is a 28-year-old construction worker diagnosed with stage I Hodgkin disease. He initially went to his health care provider because of a painful lump in his neck. He is also experiencing high fevers and weight loss. The diagnosis was confirmed in a laboratory test by the presence of Bence–Jones cells. He expresses his fears to his nurse, who tells him that Hodgkin disease is not really cancer, but it is often curable. Joe takes a leave from work and begins palliative radiation therapy.

SICKLE CELL ANEMIA REVIEW

Fill in the signs and symptoms of sickle cell anemia.

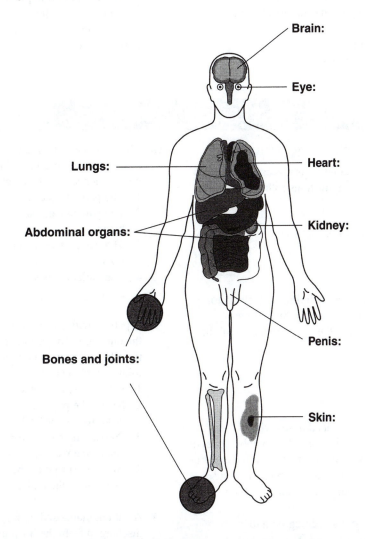

Brain:

Eye:

Lungs:

Heart:

Abdominal organs:

Kidney:

Penis:

Bones and joints:

Skin:

REVIEW QUESTIONS—CONTENT REVIEW

Choose the best answer unless directed otherwise.

1. Which of the following foods will best help provide dietary iron for a patient who has iron-deficiency anemia?
   1. Fresh fruits
   2. Lean red meats
   3. Dairy products
   4. Breads and cereals

2. A 50-year-old African American patient is diagnosed with anemia. Where can the nurse best observe for pallor?
   1. Scalp
   2. Axillae
   3. Chest
   4. Conjunctivae

3. Which of the following is an early sign of anemia?
   1. Palpitations
   2. Glossitis
   3. Pallor
   4. Weight loss

4. For which of the following problems should the nurse monitor in the patient with multiple myeloma?
   1. Uncontrolled bleeding
   2. Respiratory distress
   3. Liver engorgement
   4. Pathological fractures

5. Which of the following interventions can help minimize complications related to hypercalcemia?
   1. Encourage 3 to 4 liters of fluid daily.
   2. Have the patient cough and deep breathe every 2 hours.
   3. Place the patient on bedrest.
   4. Apply heat to painful areas.

6. A patient is admitted for a splenectomy. Why is an injection of vitamin K ordered before surgery?
   1. To correct clotting problems
   2. To promote healing
   3. To prevent postoperative infection
   4. To dry secretions

REVIEW QUESTIONS—TEST PREPARATION

Choose the best answer unless directed otherwise.

7. Which of the following conditions places a patient at risk for respiratory complications following splenectomy?
   1. A low platelet count
   2. An incision near the diaphragm
   3. Early ambulation
   4. Early discharge

8. Patients are at risk for overwhelming postsplenectomy infection following splenectomy. Which of the following symptoms alerts the nurse to this possibility?
   1. Bruising
   2. Irritability
   3. Pain
   4. Fever

9. A nurse is caring for a patient admitted with gastrointestinal tract bleeding and a hemoglobin level of 6 g/dL. The patient asks the nurse why the low hemoglobin causes shortness of breath. Which response is best?
   1. "Anemia prevents your lungs from absorbing oxygen effectively."
   2. "You do not have enough hemoglobin to carry oxygen to your tissues."
   3. "You don't have enough blood to feed your cells."
   4. "You have lost a lot of blood, and that has damaged your lungs."

10. A 27-year-old patient is admitted in sickle cell crisis. Which of the following events most likely contributed to the onset of the crisis?
    1. The patient started a new job last week.
    2. The patient walked home in a cold rain yesterday.
    3. The patient had seafood for dinner last night.
    4. The patient has not exercised for a week.

11. A patient has hand-foot syndrome related to sickle cell anemia. What findings does the nurse expect to see as the patient is examined?
    1. Unequal growth of fingers and toes
    2. Webbing between fingers and toes
    3. Purplish discoloration of hands and feet
    4. Deformities of the wrists and ankles

12. The nurse has taught a patient with thrombocytopenia how to prevent bleeding. Which of the following is the best evidence that the teaching has been effective?
    1. The patient states the importance of avoiding injury.
    2. The patient can list signs and symptoms of bleeding.
    3. The patient uses an electric razor instead of a safety razor.
    4. The patient lists symptoms that should be reported to the doctor.

13. A patient with a history of hemophilia A arrives in the emergency department with a "funny feeling" in the elbow. The patient believes he is bleeding into the joint. Which response by the nurse is correct?
    1. Palpate the patient's elbow to assess for swelling.
    2. Notify the physician immediately and expect an order for factor VIII.
    3. Prepare the patient for an x-ray examination to determine whether bleeding is occurring.
    4. Apply heat to the elbow and wait for the physician to examine the patient.

14. A patient diagnosed with lymphoma is being discharged from the hospital. Which of the following statements should the nurse include in the patient teaching? **Select all that apply.**
    1. "It is important to avoid crowds to reduce your risk of infection."
    2. "Avoid exposure to the sun, and wear sunscreen if you go outside."
    3. "It is important for you to increase your dietary intake of iron."
    4. "Your disease often affects the eyes, so television viewing should be minimized."
    5. "Be sure to wash all fruits and vegetables thoroughly before eating them."

15. What discharge teaching is most important to help the patient who has had a splenectomy prevent infection?
    1. Avoid showering for 1 week.
    2. Sleep in a semi-Fowler position.
    3. Receive a yearly flu vaccine.
    4. Stay on antibiotics for life.

CHAPTER 29

Respiratory System Function, Assessment, and Therapeutic Measures

Name:	_____
Date:	_____
Course:	_____
Instructor:	_____

AUDIO CASE STUDY

Listen to the audio case study available on Davis Edge and then answer the following questions.

Jenna Treats Mr. Jackson's Dyspnea

1. How did Jenna know Mr. Jackson was in respiratory distress?

   _____
   _____
   _____
   _____

2. What interventions did she use to help raise his oxygen saturation (Spo2) to an acceptable level?

   _____
   _____
   _____
   _____

3. Why is 90% to 92% an acceptable Spo2 in a chronic respiratory patient?

   _____
   _____
   _____
   _____

VOCABULARY

Complete the sentences with the terms provided below.

Adventitious	Barrel	Dyspnea	Thoracentesis	Tracheostomy
Apnea	Crepitus	Excursion	Tidaling	Tracheotomy

1. A patient with hypoxemia may develop shortness of breath, also called _____.

2. _____ may develop if air leaks into tissues from a chest tube site.

3. A _____ may be necessary to reduce distress from severe pleural effusion.

4. The patient with air trapping may develop a _____ -shaped chest.

5. The nurse can measure respiratory _____ to check chest expansion.

6. Crackles are an example of a/an _____ sound.

7. A patient who is choking may need an emergency _____.

8. The _____ in the water-seal chamber shows that a chest tube is intact.

9. The absence of respirations is called _____.

10. The inner cannula of a _____ tube must be removed every 8 hours for cleaning.

ANATOMY REVIEW

Number the following structures in the order in which air flows through them.

_____ Nose

_____ Trachea

_____ Secondary bronchi

_____ Primary bronchi

_____ Bronchioles

_____ Alveoli

_____ Larynx

_____ Nasopharynx

VENTILATION REVIEW

Number the events of breathing in proper sequence beginning with the medulla.

_____ The medulla generates motor impulses.

_____ The diaphragm and external intercostal muscles contract.

_____ Intrapulmonic pressure decreases.

_____ Motor impulses travel along the phrenic and intercostal nerves.

_____ The chest wall expands the parietal pleura, which expands the visceral pleura, which in turn expands the lungs.

_____ Air enters the lungs until intrapulmonic pressure equals atmospheric pressure.

ADVENTITIOUS LUNG SOUNDS

Match the adventitious lung sound to its description.

1. _____ Coarse crackles

2. _____ Fine crackles

3. _____ Wheezes

4. _____ Stridor

5. _____ Pleural friction rub

6. _____ Diminished

1. Velcro being torn apart

2. Faint lung sounds

3. Leather rubbing together

4. Loud crowing noise

5. Moist bubbling

6. High-pitched violins

CHEST DRAINAGE

Label the three chambers of the chest drainage system and explain the function of each.

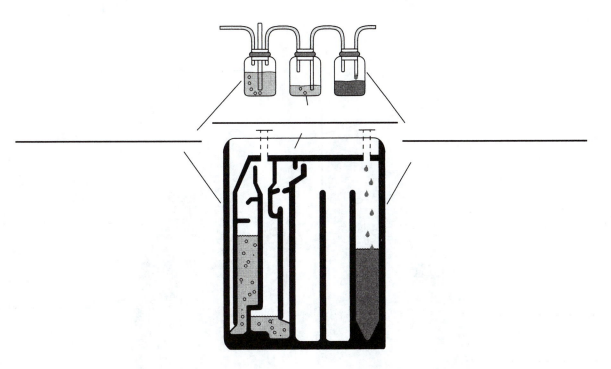

THE RESPIRATORY SYSTEM

Label the parts of the respiratory system.

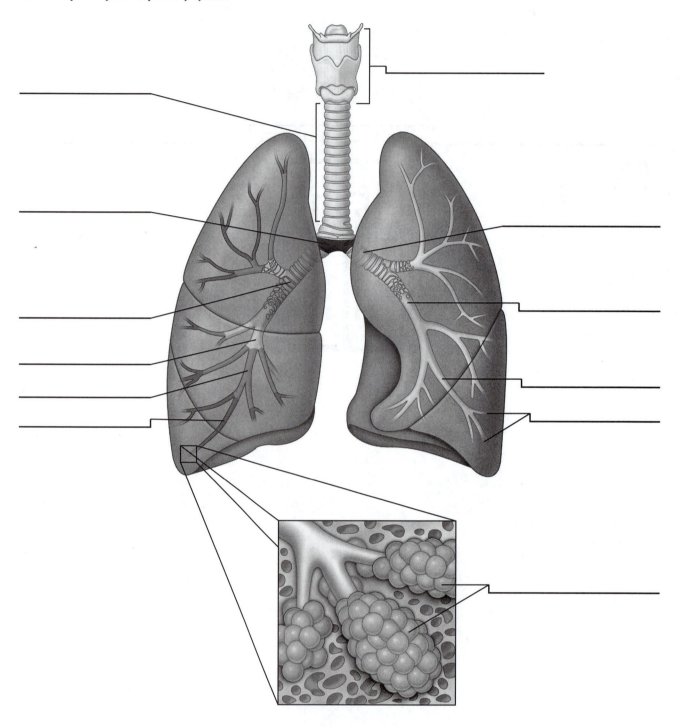

CRITICAL THINKING

Read the following case study and answer the questions.

Bill, a licensed practical nurse (LPN), is collecting admission data on Mr. Howe, who has been admitted for dyspnea and weight loss. While questioning Mr. Howe, Bill learns that he has had progressive weight loss during the past several months and that he has a productive cough. He also reports waking up at night "wringing wet," and his wife has to help him change the bed sheets.

1. What additional questions should Bill ask about Mr. Howe's cough?

   _____

   _____

   _____

2. What disorder is suggested by Mr. Howe's symptoms?

   _____

   _____

   _____

3. What diagnostic tests would you expect to be ordered?

   _____

   _____

4. Mr. Howe is scheduled for a bronchoscopy. What preprocedure care should Bill provide? Postprocedure care?

   _____

   _____

   _____

   _____

   _____

REVIEW QUESTIONS—CONTENT REVIEW

Choose the best answer unless directed otherwise.

1. Which of the following structures covers the larynx during swallowing?
   1. Hyoid cartilage
   2. Vocal cords
   3. Soft palate
   4. Epiglottis

2. Where are the respiratory centers located in the brain?
   1. Cerebral cortex and cerebellum
   2. Medulla and pons
   3. Hypothalamus and cerebral cortex
   4. Hypothalamus and temporal lobes

3. What is the purpose of the serous fluid between the pleural membranes?
   1. Enhance exchange of gases
   2. Facilitate coughing
   3. Destroy pathogens
   4. Prevent friction

4. Within the alveoli, surface tension is decreased and inflation is possible because of the presence of which substance?
   1. Tissue fluid
   2. Surfactant
   3. Pulmonary blood
   4. Mucus

5. What is the function of the nasal mucosa?
   1. Assist with gas exchange
   2. Sweep mucus and pathogens to the trachea
   3. Warm and moisten the incoming air
   4. Increase the oxygen content of the air

6. Deteriorating cilia in the respiratory tract predispose older adults to which of the following problems?
   1. Chronic hypoxia
   2. Pulmonary hypertension
   3. Respiratory infection
   4. Decreased ventilation

7. Which of the following adventitious lung sounds is a violin-like sound?
   1. Crackles
   2. Wheezes
   3. Friction rub
   4. Crepitus

8. The purpose of pursed-lip breathing is to promote which of the following?
   1. Carbon dioxide excretion
   2. Carbon dioxide retention
   3. Oxygen excretion
   4. Oxygen retention

REVIEW QUESTIONS—TEST PREPARATION

Choose the best answer unless directed otherwise.

9. A nurse enters the room of a patient with chronic lung disease. The patient has removed the oxygen cannula, and it is lying on the bed. The patient does not appear to be in any distress. The pulse oximeter shows an oxygen saturation of 79%. Which of the following actions should the nurse take?
   1. Call the registered nurse STAT.
   2. Put the oxygen cannula back on the patient.
   3. Administer a nebulized mist treatment.
   4. No action is necessary; the patient is not in distress.

10. A patient hospitalized with a right-sided pleural effusion calls the nurse and reports feeling short of breath. Which of the following positions should the nurse suggest?
   1. Prone
   2. Supine with head on pillow
   3. Trendelenburg
   4. Side lying with good lung dependent

11. The nurse is caring for a patient with a transtracheal catheter. Which of the following would the nurse expect to be included in the plan of care?
   1. Assist with cleaning the catheter two to three times a day.
   2. Provide supplemental oxygen via mask at all times.
   3. Help remove the catheter at night for sleeping.
   4. Assist to connect the catheter to a humidification source.

12. The spouse of a patient with cystic fibrosis has been taught how to perform chest physiotherapy. The spouse asks the nurse to explain why this must be done. Which of the following responses is best?
   1. "It helps strengthen chest muscles."
   2. "It humidifies thick respiratory secretions."
   3. "It promotes lung expansion."
   4. "It helps him expectorate secretions."

13. The nurse is assessing a patient with a chest drainage system. What data should be collected? **Select all that apply.**
   1. Auscultate lung sounds.
   2. Remove chest dressing to inspect the insertion site.
   3. Palpate for crepitus.
   4. Check all tubing for kinks or breaks.
   5. Check fluid levels in drainage system.

14. Mark the chamber on the chest drainage system that prevents air from being reintroduced into the chest.

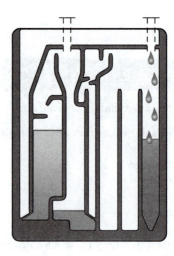

CHAPTER 30
Nursing Care of Patients With Upper Respiratory Tract Disorders

Name: _____

Date: _____

Course: _____

Instructor: _____

AUDIO CASE STUDY

Maxine's Grandpa Has the Flu

1. What symptoms of influenza did Maxine's grandpa exhibit?

_____

_____

_____

_____

_____

2. Why are older patients more at risk for complications of flu?

_____

_____

_____

_____

_____

3. What can you teach your patients to help them avoid contracting the flu?

_____

_____

_____

_____

_____

VOCABULARY

Unscramble the letters of the following words to fill in the blanks in the statements below.

hiitsrin   aadihpysg

pixessait   daxueet

laiohnpstry   cayetorlmyng

1. Surgical removal of the voice box is called a _____.
2. A nosebleed is called _____.
3. _____ is the term used to describe drainage or pus.
4. A "nose job" is called _____.
5. Difficulty swallowing is called _____.
6. _____ is the correct term for a runny nose.

CRITICAL THINKING: NASAL SURGERY

Read the following case study and answer the questions.

Mr. Jones had a broken nose as a young man and now has a deviated nasal septum. He undergoes nasoseptoplasty for a deviated nasal septum.

1. After surgery, you note that Mr. Jones is swallowing repeatedly while he sleeps. What do you do?

   _____

   _____

   _____

   _____

2. Before discharging Mr. Jones, you explain to him that he should not do anything that can increase bleeding, such as sneezing, coughing, or straining to have a bowel movement. He says, "How can I avoid doing those things? It sounds impossible." How do you respond?

   _____

   _____

   _____

   _____

3. Mr. Jones asks if he can use aspirin for pain. What do you say?

   _____

   _____

   _____

   _____

CRITICAL THINKING: INFLUENZA

Read the following case study and answer the questions.

Your 38-year-old neighbor calls and describes symptoms of influenza. He is feverish and tired, and has a sore throat and headache. You advise him to go to the urgent care center. The center does a throat culture and determines that the infection is viral, most likely the flu. Your neighbor is encouraged to drink fluids and take acetaminophen.

1. Why didn't the health care provider order antibiotics? _____

   _____

   _____

2. How will fluids help? _____

   _____

   _____

3. When should the acetaminophen be taken? _____

   _____

   _____

4. Your neighbor's wife develops the same symptoms. Is it necessary to take her to the urgent care center?

   _____

   _____

   _____

5. Your neighbor's older grandmother was visiting when your neighbor first developed symptoms. She now thinks she has caught the flu, and her chest hurts. She asks what she should do. What should you tell her?

   _____

   _____

   _____

REVIEW QUESTIONS—CONTENT REVIEW

Choose the best answer unless directed otherwise.

1. When evaluating the effectiveness of nursing interventions for sinusitis pain, which data does the nurse collect?
   1. White blood cell count
   2. Amount and color of sinus drainage
   3. Capillary refill
   4. Pain level on a 0 to 10 scale

2. Why are narcotics given in lower doses for pain to the patient who has had a laryngectomy?
   1. They depress the respiratory rate and cough reflex.
   2. They increase respiratory tract secretions.
   3. They have a tendency to cause stomal edema.
   4. They can cause addiction.

3. Which of the following are early symptoms of laryngeal cancer?
   1. Anemia and fatigue
   2. Crackles and stridor
   3. A noticeable lump in the neck
   4. Dysphagia or hoarseness

4. A patient visits a nurse practitioner after having a cold for a week. The patient is now experiencing a severe headache and fever. The nurse practitioner diagnoses a sinus infection. Which of the following additional symptoms is the patient likely to exhibit?
   1. Facial tenderness
   2. Chest pain
   3. Photophobia
   4. Ear drainage

REVIEW QUESTIONS—TEST PREPARATION

Choose the best answer unless directed otherwise.

5. Which of the following recommendations can the nurse make to increase comfort for a patient experiencing sinusitis? **Select all that apply.**
   1. Coughing and deep breathing
   2. Sinus irrigation
   3. Hot moist packs
   4. Room humidifier
   5. Percussion and postural drainage
   6. Semi-Fowler position

6. Place in correct order of priority the following four nursing actions for a patient who has just had a laryngectomy.
   1. Assist with ambulation.
   2. Set up a visit from a well-adjusted patient who has had a laryngectomy.
   3. Maintain a patent airway.
   4. Control postoperative pain.

7. The nurse teaches a patient how to live with a new tracheostomy. Which of the following instructions is appropriate?
   1. "Never suction your tracheostomy. You might damage your trachea."
   2. "You should not feel bad about the tracheostomy—you should feel lucky to be alive."
   3. "Be sure to protect your tracheostomy from pollutants such as powders or hair."
   4. "Your tracheostomy will be cleaned each time you visit your doctor."

8. A 17-year-old student enters the emergency department with a nosebleed that won't stop. The nurse should assist the patient to assume which of the following positions?
   1. Lying down with feet elevated
   2. Sitting up with neck extended
   3. Lying down with a small pillow under the head
   4. Sitting up leaning slightly forward

9. The health care provider orders local application of phenylephrine solution to treat a nosebleed. The patient asks how this will help. Which of the following responses by the nurse is best?
   1. "It will raise your blood pressure, which is necessary because of blood loss."
   2. "It will dilate your bronchioles and make your breathing easier."
   3. "It will help your blood to clot to reduce bleeding."
   4. "It will constrict your vessels and slow down the bleeding."

10. A nurse is providing community education related to West Nile virus. Which of the following statements by a participant indicates that teaching has been effective?
    1. "I've eliminated all pork from my diet."
    2. "I will not travel outside the United States."
    3. "I will wear mosquito repellent when I am outdoors."
    4. "I will avoid bird and bat droppings."

CHAPTER 31
Nursing Care of Patients With Lower Respiratory Tract Disorders

Name: _____

Date: _____

Course: _____

Instructor: _____

AUDIO CASE STUDY

Listen to the audio case study available on Davis Edge and then answer the following questions.

Jack Has Emphysema and COPD

1. What are the pathophysiologies of chronic obstructive pulmonary disease (COPD) and emphysema?

_____

_____

_____

_____

_____

_____

2. How does pursed lip breathing promote carbon dioxide elimination in COPD?

_____

_____

_____

3. Will Jack's son's lungs return to normal once he quits smoking?

_____

_____

_____

RESPIRATORY MEDICATIONS

Match the medication with its action.

1. _____ Prednisone

2. _____ Albuterol (Ventolin)

3. _____ Tiotropium (Spiriva)

4. _____ Beclomethasone (Beclovent)

5. _____ Guaifenesin (Mucinex)

6. _____ Zafirlukast (Accolate)

7. _____ Codeine

1. Expectorant

2. Anti-inflammatory steroid (oral)

3. Antileukotrienes

4. Short-acting beta-agonist bronchodilator

5. Anticholinergic bronchodilator

6. Inhaled corticosteroid

7. Antitussive

CRITICAL THINKING

Read the following case study and answer the questions.

Edith is a 56-year-old homemaker admitted to the hospital with emphysema and acute dyspnea. She is a smoker with a 48-pack-year history.

1. What data do you collect for Edith's admission database?

2. What does a 48-pack-year history mean?

3. Explain the pathophysiology involved in emphysema. How does the disease cause dyspnea?

4. What do you expect Edith's lungs to sound like when you auscultate?

5. Why is it important for Edith to maintain her peripheral capillary oxygen saturation (Spo_2) between 88% and 92% instead of at the normal level of 95% or more?

6. Why might Edith be at risk for a pneumothorax?

_____

_____

_____

_____

7. What position will help Edith's shortness of breath? Why?

_____

_____

_____

_____

8. How can you encourage Edith to stop smoking?

_____

_____

_____

_____

_____

REVIEW QUESTIONS—CONTENT REVIEW

Choose the best answer unless directed otherwise.

1. What is the purpose of corticosteroid treatment in lung disease?
   1. Dry up secretions
   2. Treat the infection that causes an exacerbation
   3. Improve the oxygen-carrying capacity of hemoglobin
   4. Reduce airway inflammation

2. What is the desired peripheral capillary oxygen saturation (SpO_2) level in the patient with chronic obstructive pulmonary disease?
   1. 95% to 100%
   2. 92% to 95%
   3. 88% to 92%
   4. 85% to 88%

3. Which of the following medications can be used to quickly reduce shortness of breath in a crisis situation for a patient with end-stage respiratory disease?
   1. Oral cortisone
   2. Intramuscular meperidine (Demerol)
   3. Intravenous morphine
   4. Intravenous propranolol (Inderal)

4. Which of the following risk factors presents the greatest threat for respiratory disease?
   1. Smoking
   2. High-fat diet
   3. Exposure to radiation
   4. Alcohol consumption

REVIEW QUESTIONS—TEST PREPARATION

Choose the best answer unless directed otherwise.

5. A patient with pneumonia has an oxygen saturation result of 86%. Which of the following actions by the nurse is best?
   1. Contact the registered nurse or health care provider for an order for oxygen.
   2. No action necessary; this is a normal peripheral capillary oxygen saturation (SpO_2).
   3. Call the respiratory therapist STAT for assistance.
   4. Walk the patient in the hall and recheck the oxygen saturation.

6. Which as-needed medication should be administered first in the patient with acute asthma symptoms?
   1. Albuterol (Proventil) inhaler
   2. Triamcinolone acetonide (Azmacort) inhaler
   3. Fluticasone and salmeterol (Advair) inhaler
   4. Montelukast (Singulair) orally

7. Which nursing interventions are important for the patient who is unable to cough up thick secretions? **Select all that apply.**
    1. Assist the patient to ambulate regularly.
    2. Place a cool steamer in the patient's room.
    3. Administer antitussive medication as ordered.
    4. Guide the patient in coughing and deep breathing.
    5. Teach the patient relaxation exercises.

8. A patient asks how to avoid lung cancer. Which of the following should the nurse include in the patient teaching? **Select all that apply.**
    1. Live in a cold climate.
    2. Stop smoking.
    3. Avoid exposure to passive smoke.
    4. Avoid air pollution.
    5. Avoid crowded living conditions.
    6. Consume a diet high in fruits and vegetables.

9. A patient with a new diagnosis of small cell lung cancer decides to have radiation therapy. Which of the following expectations of this treatment is most appropriate?
    1. Complete cure of the cancer
    2. Increased comfort
    3. Prevention of the need for oxygen
    4. Prevention of cancer spread

10. A newly diagnosed patient asks the nurse to explain asthma. Which of the following explanations by the nurse is correct?
    1. "Your airways are inflamed and spastic."
    2. "You have fluid in your lungs that is causing shortness of breath."
    3. "Your airways are stretched and nonfunctional."
    4. "You have a low-grade infection that keeps your bronchial tree irritated."

11. Which of the following is the best explanation of emphysema for a newly diagnosed patient?
    1. "You have inflamed bronchioles, which causes a lot of secretions."
    2. "The blood vessels that supply your lungs are damaged, so you can't absorb oxygen."
    3. "Your lungs have lost some of their elasticity, and air gets trapped."
    4. "You have large dilated sacs of sputum in your lungs."

12. How can the nurse monitor effectiveness of therapy for the patient with a pneumothorax and a chest drainage system?
    1. Palpate for crepitus.
    2. Auscultate lung sounds.
    3. Document color and amount of sputum.
    4. Monitor suction level.

13. The nurse is collecting data on a patient with suspected left lower lobe pneumonia. Mark the area where the nurse would expect to hear crackles when auscultating the chest.

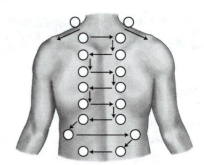

CHAPTER 32

Gastrointestinal, Hepatobiliary, and Pancreatic Systems Function, Assessment, and Therapeutic Measures

Name:
Date:
Course:
Instructor:

AUDIO CASE STUDY

Listen to the audio case study available on Davis Edge and then answer the following questions.

Grace and Enteral Feedings

1. What care for feeding tubes and enteral tube–feeding systems was used to prevent complications?

_____

_____

_____

_____

2. How was placement of the feeding tube verified?

_____

_____

3. What positioning was used during the feedings?

_____

_____

4. What is done for pneumonia prevention during the feedings?

_____

_____

_____

FUNCTIONS OF THE GASTROINTESTINAL SYSTEM

Fill in the blanks with the appropriate parts of the gastrointestinal (GI) system.

1. The lower _____ sphincter prevents backup of stomach contents into the esophagus.

2. The _____ valve prevents backup of fecal material from the large intestine into the small intestine.

3. The _____ sphincter prevents backup of duodenal contents into the stomach.

4. The absorption of most of the end products of digestion occurs in the _____ intestine.

5. The digestion of protein begins in the _____ .

6. Water and the vitamins produced by the normal flora are absorbed in the _____ intestine.

7. The _____ intestine is the site of action of bile and pancreatic enzymes.

8. The passageway for food into the stomach from the mouth is the _____ .

9. Voluntary control of defecation is provided by the _____ anal sphincter.

10. The watery secretion that permits taste and swallowing is produced by the _____ glands.

11. The process of mechanical digestion is accomplished by the _____ and _____ in the mouth.

12. The structures in the small intestine that contain capillaries and lacteals for absorption are the _____ .

13. The part of the colon that contracts in the defecation reflex is the _____ .

14. The digestive function of the liver is the production of _____ by the hepatocytes.

STRUCTURES OF THE GASTROINTESTINAL SYSTEM

Label the following structures.

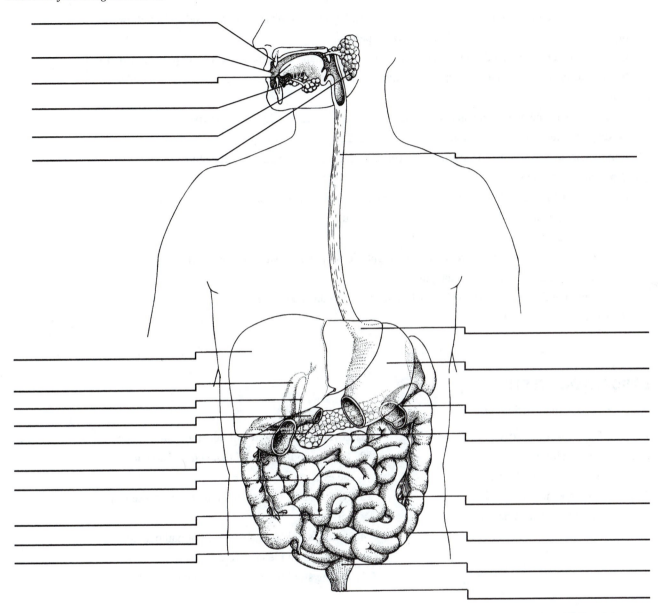

VOCABULARY

Unscramble the letters to identify the word described by the definition.

1. Flexible or rigid device consisting of a tube and optical system for observing the inside of a hollow organ or cavity. _____ donscepeo

2. Gurgling and clicking heard over the abdomen caused by air and fluid movement from peristaltic action that can be classified as normal, hypoactive, hyperactive, or absent. _____ wlebo onudss

3. Examination of the colon with an endoscope. _____ locnooscypo

4. Feeding via a tube placed in the stomach. _____ gvaaeg

5. Immovable accumulation of feces in the bowels. _____ mipcaitno

6. Blood not visible in feces. _____ ccoltu

7. Device consisting of a fluorescent screen that makes the shadows of objects interposed between the tube and the screen visible. _____ ulfroocspeo

8. Fatty stools. _____ estaotrhrae

9. A test performed to measure secretions of hydrochloric acid and pepsin in the stomach. _____ stgairc naayliss

10. Examination of the stomach and abdominal cavity by use of an endoscope. _____ stgarsopcoy

---

LABORATORY TESTS

Match the test with its definition.

1. _____ Stool for fat (lipids)
2. _____ Stool cultures
3. _____ Stool for occult blood
4. _____ Carcinoembryonic antigen
5. _____ Stool for ova and parasites

1. Levels may indicate colorectal or other cancer.
2. Testing stool for blood that is not visible to the eye.
3. Testing stool for intestinal infections caused by parasites.
4. Testing stool for the presence of pathogenic organisms in the GI tract.
5. Testing stool for excessive amounts of fat.

BOWEL PREPARATION

Circle the eight errors in the following paragraph, and insert the correct information.

A stomach preparation is required for several procedures that visualize the lower bowel. This preparation is important for effective test results. An incomplete bowel preparation may prevent the test from being done or cause the need for it to be repeated. This can result in the patient's early discharge and cost savings. The patient usually receives a soft diet 24 hours before the test. A laxative may be given. Enemas may be given once. Young or debilitated patients should be carefully monitored during the administration of multiple enemas, which can fatigue the patient and increase electrolytes. In patients with bleeding or constipation, the bowel preparation may not be ordered by the health care provider.

PANCREAS

Identify the pancreatic enzyme by its function.

1. Digests polypeptides to short chains of amino acids.

_____

2. Digests emulsified fats to fatty acids and glycerol.

_____

3. Digests starch to maltose.

_____

LIVER

Fill in the blanks with the appropriate words.

1. Liver or gallbladder disease may cause pale or _____ -colored stools.

2. Liver disease may cause _____ disorders.

3. A liver scan records the amount of _____ material taken up by the liver to form a composite "picture" of the liver.

4. After a liver biopsy, the patient lies on the right side for the first _____ hours.

5. After a liver biopsy, nursing care focuses on monitoring for _____.

CRITICAL THINKING

Read the following case study and answer the questions.

Mrs. Davis is a 41-year-old schoolteacher who is admitted to your unit with esophageal cancer. Her health care provider orders enteral nutrition through her gastrostomy tube.

1. Before beginning the feeding, what action should you take for patient-centered care?

_____

_____

2. How will you verify the correct placement of the gastrostomy tube?

_____

_____

3. How should the patient be positioned during the feedings? Why?

_____

_____

4. What actions should you take to set up the feeding safely?

_____

_____

_____

_____

5. Why should a controller pump be used for a continuous feeding?

_____

_____

_____

6. What action can you take to prevent patient dehydration? What health care team member should you consult for this?

_____

_____

7. Describe tube flushing. What are two benefits of tube flushing?

_____

_____

_____

_____

REVIEW QUESTIONS—CONTENT REVIEW

Choose the best answer unless directed otherwise.

1. Which of the following structures are connected by the ileocecal valve?
   1. Duodenum to the stomach
   2. Colon to the small intestine
   3. Stomach to the esophagus
   4. Ileum to the jejunum

2. Mechanical digestion in the stomach is accomplished by which of the following structures?
   1. Mucosa
   2. Smooth muscle layers
   3. Striated muscle layers
   4. Gastric glands

3. Gastric juice contributes to the digestion of which of the following types of nutrients?
   1. Proteins
   2. Fats
   3. Starch

4. The enzymes of the small intestine contribute to the digestion of which of the following types of nutrients?
   1. Starch
   2. Fats
   3. Disaccharides

5. Which of the following structures carries bile and pancreatic juices to the duodenum?
   1. Pancreatic duct
   2. Cystic duct
   3. Hepatic duct
   4. Common bile duct

6. Which of the following is a function of the liver?
   1. Synthesis of plasma proteins
   2. Elimination of carbohydrates
   3. Concentration of bile
   4. Secretion of cholecystokinin

7. Which of the following diagnostic procedures on stool specimens must the nurse collect using sterile technique?
   1. Stool for ova and parasites
   2. Stool for occult blood
   3. Stool for culture
   4. Stool for lipids

8. Which of the following colors would the nurse recognize as an expected finding for the patient's stools immediately after a barium enema?
   1. Brown
   2. Black
   3. Green
   4. White

REVIEW QUESTIONS—TEST PREPARATION

Choose the best answer unless directed otherwise.

9. The nurse evaluates the patient as understanding the primary reason that food and fluids are held until the gag reflex returns after an esophagogastroduo-denoscopy procedure if the patient states which of these?
   1. "To rest the vocal cords."
   2. "To prevent aspiration."
   3. "To keep the throat dry."
   4. "To prevent vomiting."

10. What action should the nurse take prior to initiating an enteral feeding using a newly inserted nasogastric feeding tube?
   1. Auscultate bowel sounds.
   2. Flush the feeding tube.
   3. Review chest x-ray results.
   4. Review abdominal x-ray results.

11. The nurse auscultates the patient's abdomen and finds it to be silent. The nurse would document the bowel sounds findings as which of these?
   1. Absent
   2. Hyperactive
   3. Hypoactive
   4. Normal

12. When teaching patients about diagnostic procedures, the nurse would include food and fluid restrictions prior to the test for which of these? **Select all that apply.**
   1. Barium swallow
   2. Flat plate of the abdomen
   3. Esophagogastroduodenoscopy
   4. Magnetic resonance imaging
   5. Endoscopic retrograde cholangiopancreatography
   6. Barium enema

13. The nurse would evaluate the patient as understanding teaching if the patient replied that which of the following can occur following a barium swallow? **Select all that apply.**
   1. Dysphagia
   2. Constipation
   3. Diarrhea
   4. Pain
   5. White stool

14. What actions can the nurse take to ensure patient safety when providing an enteral feeding? **Select all that apply.**
    1. Use adequate room lighting.
    2. Trace all lines back to their origins.
    3. Check connections during patient handoff.
    4. Reconnect a patient's tubing to assist another nurse.
    5. Route all tubes in the same direction.
    6. Do not interfere with equipment safety features.

15. The nurse is collecting data from a patient with ascites to identify if the ascites has increased. Mark the area where the nurse would obtain this measurement.

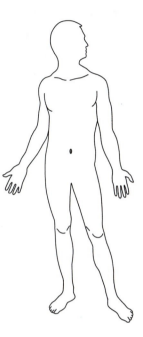

CHAPTER 33
Nursing Care of Patients With Upper Gastrointestinal Disorders

Name:	
Date:	
Course:	
Instructor:	

AUDIO CASE STUDY

Listen to the audio case study available on Davis Edge and then answer the following questions.

Darnell and Peptic Ulcer Disease

1. What was discovered in 1982 that is the cause of most peptic ulcers?

_____

_____

_____

_____

_____

2. What are the symptoms of a gastric ulcer?

_____

_____

_____

_____

_____

3. What is treatment for *Helicobacter pylori*?

_____

_____

_____

_____

_____

VOCABULARY

Unscramble the letters to identify a word described by the definition.

1. The most common cause of peptic ulcers whose discovery revolutionized treatment and cure of most peptic ulcers. _____ lehicbocatre ypoilr

2. Loss of appetite. _____ noraxeai

3. Inflammation of the stomach. _____ sagrtisti

4. Small, white, painful ulcers that appear on the inner cheeks, lips, gums, tongue, palate, and pharynx. _____ hpatouhs tsoamtisti

5. Term for weight loss surgery from the Greek *baros*. _____ arbairtci

6. Excessive fat in the stools. _____ teasrroteha

7. Surgical removal of the stomach. _____ gtrasetcmyo

8. 20% to 30% over average weight for age, sex, and height. _____ boesiyt

9. Condition in which the stomach may protrude above the diaphragm. _____ ihaatl erhian

10. Following surgical removal of part of the stomach, reanastomosis of the remaining portion to the proximal jejunum. _____ satgorjujeonsotym

---

GASTRITIS

Match the description with the type of gastritis associated with it.

1. _____ Heartburn or indigestion

2. _____ Autoimmune gastritis

3. _____ Often caused by overeating

4. _____ Bacteria *Helicobacter pylori*

5. _____ Difficulty in absorbing vitamin B_{12}

6. _____ Can lead to peritonitis

7. _____ Can be treated with antibiotics

8. _____ Treatment is to avoid alcohol and irritating foods

1. Acute gastritis

2. Chronic gastritis type A

3. Chronic gastritis type B

PEPTIC ULCER DISEASE

Circle the seven errors in the following paragraph and insert the correct information.

Most peptic ulcers are caused by stress. Peptic ulcers are commonly found in the sigmoid colon. Symptoms of peptic ulcers include burning and a gnawing pain in the chest. With a duodenal ulcer, there is pain and discomfort with a full stomach, which may be relieved by avoiding food. Peptic ulcers cannot be cured. Medication treatment for peptic ulcers caused by *H. pylori* should include anticoagulants as indicated.

GASTRECTOMY

Label the structures as they appear following various types of gastric surgery.

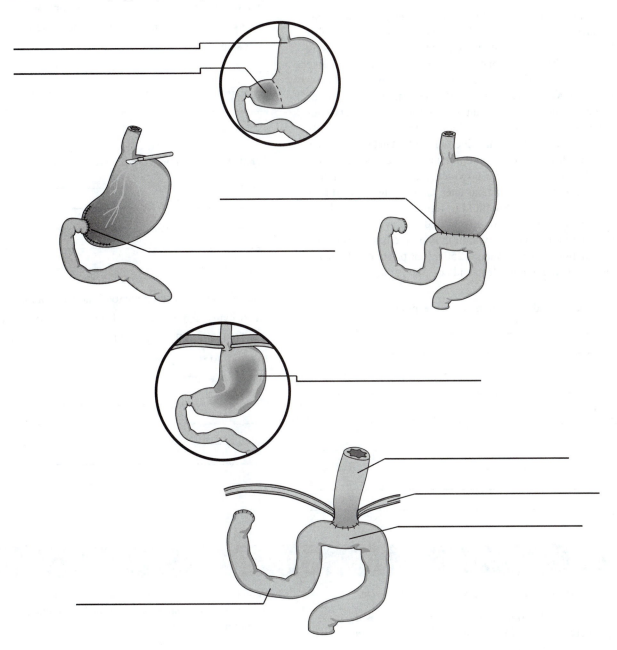

CRITICAL THINKING

Read the following case study and answer the questions.

Mrs. Sheffield has just returned from surgery. She had a gastroduodenostomy (Billroth I) procedure. She has a nasogastric (NG) tube, 1,000 mL of lactated Ringer solution infusing at 100 mL/hr via intravenous (IV) route, and a Foley catheter. She is nil per os (NPO). Her vital signs are stable: blood pressure 118/90 mm Hg, pulse 80 beats per minute, respirations 16 per minute, and temperature 98°F (36.6°C). Her abdominal dressing is clean, dry, and intact. She is drowsy but easily aroused. After getting Mrs. Sheffield settled in bed, the nurse connects her NG tube to intermittent low-wall suction as ordered by her health care provider (HCP) and adds another blanket for warmth. An hour later, the nursing assistant tells the nurse that Mrs. Sheffield is vomiting bright red blood. The nurse goes to her room and finds her lying on her side propped up on one arm vomiting into an emesis basin. Her NG suction catheter contains 250 mL of bright red drainage. Her dressing remains clean and dry. She is diaphoretic.

1. What should be the nurse's first response?

   _____

   _____

   _____

   _____

2. What is the nurse's next action?

   _____

   _____

   _____

   _____

3. Vital signs are now blood pressure 86/60 mm Hg, pulse 96 beats per minute, respirations 24 per minute, and temperature 97.6°F (36.4°C). What is the nurse's analysis of the new data? What are the nurse's next steps?

   _____

   _____

   _____

   _____

4. What should the nurse tell the HCP?

   _____

   _____

   _____

   _____

   _____

5. The HCP orders a stat hematocrit and hemoglobin, electrolytes, and oxygen at 2 L/min via nasal cannula. The HCP also tells the nurse to get Mrs. Sheffield ready to return to surgery. What are the nurse's priority nursing actions?

   _____

   _____

   _____

   _____

   _____

REVIEW QUESTIONS—CONTENT REVIEW

Choose the best answer unless directed otherwise.

1. Which of the following surgical procedures is the most likely treatment for a patient with gastric cancer?
   1. Gastrectomy
   2. Gastric stapling
   3. Gastroplasty
   4. Gastrorrhaphy

2. Which of the following does the nurse understand is a sign or symptom of oral cancer?
   1. Painless ulcer
   2. White painful ulcers
   3. Feeling of fullness
   4. Heartburn

3. Which of the following procedures does the nurse understand is done palliatively for the dysphagia that occurs in inoperable esophageal cancer?
   1. Gastrectomy
   2. Esophageal dilation
   3. Radical neck dissection
   4. Modified neck dissection

REVIEW QUESTIONS—TEST PREPARATION

Choose the best answer unless directed otherwise.

4. A patient is diagnosed with aphthous stomatitis (canker sore). Which nursing action should the nurse implement?
   1. Explain not to brush teeth until the sore has healed.
   2. Encourage patient to use a mouthwash four times a day.
   3. Apply acyclovir ointment to sore for pain relief.
   4. Teach patient to apply topical tetracycline several times a day to the sore.

5. A patient is admitted with chronic gastritis type B. Which of the following signs and symptoms would the nurse anticipate finding?
   1. Anorexia
   2. Dysphagia
   3. Diarrhea
   4. Feeling of fullness

6. An asymptomatic patient is admitted with gastric bleeding. For which of the following signs or symptoms of severe gastric bleeding should the nurse monitor? **Select all that apply.**
   1. Restlessness
   2. Diaphoresis
   3. Bounding pulse
   4. Hypotension
   5. Confusion

7. A patient had a gastrectomy 2 months ago and is being seen in the clinic for greasy stools and frequent bowel movements. After the patient's surgical recovery and current eating habits are identified, which type of diet would be most appropriate for the nurse to teach the patient to use?
   1. Soft diet
   2. High-carbohydrate diet
   3. Low-fat diet
   4. Pureed diet

8. During a visit with the health care provider, the patient asks for guidance in losing some weight. The patient is currently 310 pounds with a height of 5 foot 7 inches. When contributing to the plan of care, the nurse would recognize that the initial treatment for obesity would include which of these? **Select all that apply.**
   1. Biofeedback
   2. Calorie restriction
   3. Counseling
   4. Healthy diet
   5. Exercise
   6. Fasting

9. A patient has been diagnosed with a hiatal hernia. The patient has heartburn and occasional regurgitation. Which intervention should the nurse teach the patient to reduce the symptoms?
   1. Eat small, frequent meals.
   2. Recline for 1 hour after meals.
   3. Sleep flat without a pillow.
   4. Eat a bedtime snack.

10. A patient is having an acute episode of gastric bleeding. The health care provider orders 1,000 mL of 0.9% normal saline via intravenous route, a complete blood count, a nasogastric tube to low-wall suction, and oxygen by nasal cannula. Which order should the nurse perform first?
    1. Administer 1,000 mL of 0.9% normal saline.
    2. Draw blood for a complete blood count.
    3. Insert a nasogastric tube.
    4. Apply oxygen by nasal cannula.

11. A patient is taught preventive measures for gastroesophageal reflux disease. Which statement by the patient indicates that teaching has been effective?
    1. "I need to eat large meals."
    2. "I will sleep without pillows."
    3. "I need to lie down for 2 hours after each meal."
    4. "I will identify foods that cause discomfort."

12. The nurse is collecting data on a patient who recently returned from surgery after fundoplication. Which symptom is essential to report to the health care provider?
    1. Nausea
    2. Pain rated as 4 out of 10
    3. Dysphagia
    4. Thirst

13. The nurse is caring for a patient who has an emesis with a coffee ground appearance. Mark the area that is producing the coffee ground appearance.

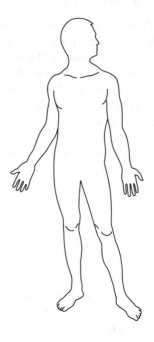

CHAPTER 34
Nursing Care of Patients With Lower Gastrointestinal Disorders

Name: _____

Date: _____

Course: _____

Instructor: _____

AUDIO CASE STUDY

Listen to the audio case study available on Davis Edge and then answer the following questions.

Tara and Gastrointestinal Bleeding

1. What was the cause of Mrs. Kirk's gastrointestinal (GI) bleeding?

_____

_____

_____

_____

_____

2. What symptoms did Mrs. Kirk have during GI bleeding?

_____

_____

_____

_____

_____

3. What treatment was ordered for Mrs. Kirk?

_____

_____

_____

_____

_____

VOCABULARY

Match the vocabulary word to the correct definition.

1. _____ Appendicitis
2. _____ Colectomy
3. _____ Colitis
4. _____ Colostomy
5. _____ Diverticulosis
6. _____ Fistula
7. _____ Hernia
8. _____ Ileostomy
9. _____ Intussusception
10. _____ Melena
11. _____ Peritonitis
12. _____ Volvulus

1. Outpouchings in colon
2. Inflammation of colon
3. Telescoping of the bowel
4. Tunnel connection between bowel and another organ
5. Blood in stool
6. Twisting of bowel
7. Inflammation or infection of peritoneum
8. Bulging of abdominal contents through abdominal wall
9. Diversion of small bowel through abdominal wall
10. Removal of large bowel
11. Diversion of large bowel through abdominal wall
12. Inflamed appendix

OSTOMIES

Circle the four errors in each one of the following paragraphs and insert the correct information.

1. Michelle Braun is a 16-year-old with ulcerative colitis. She is taking cortisone. She is on a high-residue diet. She has just been admitted to the hospital for a colectomy and elective loop ostomy. The nurse monitors her intake and output, daily weights, and electrolytes. The nurse also monitors for signs of inflammation in her joints, skin, and other parts of her body. The nurse teaches her to restrict fluids following surgery to limit the number of stools she has daily.

2. James Key is a 46-year-old with a new sigmoid colostomy. Following surgery, the nurse monitors his stoma each shift to ensure that it remains gray and moist. The nurse explains that the stool will be semiformed and that he will have to irrigate his ostomy every 1 to 2 days to have bowel movements. The nurse contacts the dietitian to provide a list of the high-fiber foods that he should eat.

CRITICAL THINKING

Read the following case study and answer the questions.

Mrs. Millie Hendricks is a 90-year-old resident in a long-term care facility. Mrs. Hendricks has a history of severe osteoarthritis, and she has no teeth but is otherwise quite healthy. She normally has a bowel movement every other day but has occasional constipation, which she takes care of herself by requesting a dose of Milk of Magnesia. Today when the nurse brings Mrs. Hendricks's medications to her, she says, "I think I need a second dose of that Milk of Magnesia. My bowels haven't moved in 3 days." The nurse looks at the medication administration record and finds as needed (prn) orders for Milk of Magnesia (magnesium hydroxide mixture), psyllium (Metamucil), senna (Senokot), or a tap water enema.

1. What should the nurse do before administering more medication?

_____
_____
_____
_____

2. What factors most likely led to Mrs. Hendricks's constipation?

_____
_____
_____
_____

3. What will happen if Mrs. Hendricks's bowels do not move today?

_____

_____

_____

_____

4. What nondrug interventions will help Mrs. Hendricks move her bowels?

_____

_____

_____

_____

_____

5. After Mrs. Hendricks's bowels have moved, what measures can be instituted to prevent constipation next time?

_____

_____

_____

_____

_____

_____

_____

REVIEW QUESTIONS—CONTENT REVIEW

Choose the best answer unless directed otherwise.

1. Which of these differentiates diverticulitis from diverticulosis? **Select all that apply.**
   1. Presence of weakness in bowel wall
   2. Presence of outpouchings on bowel mucous membrane
   3. Presence of inflammation and infection
   4. Lack of symptoms
   5. Involves the large intestine

2. A pattern of alternating constipation and diarrhea is most characteristic of which of the following gastrointestinal tract disorders?
   1. Crohn disease
   2. Ulcerative colitis
   3. Irritable bowel syndrome
   4. Large-bowel obstruction

3. Which of the following drugs would the nurse expect to be prescribed for a woman with irritable bowel syndrome and constipation? **Select all that apply.**
   1. Desipramine (Norpramin)
   2. Dicyclomine (Bentyl)
   3. Fluoxetine (Prozac)
   4. Hyoscyamine (Levbid)
   5. Nortriptyline (Pamelor)
   6. Paroxetine hydrochloride (Paxil)

4. Which of the following foods might a patient with diverticulitis have been instructed to avoid, even though this has not been proven to prevent diverticulitis? **Select all that apply.**
   1. Apples
   2. Dairy products
   3. Peanuts
   4. Red meat
   5. Raspberries
   6. Whole grains

REVIEW QUESTIONS—TEST PREPARATION

Choose the best answer unless directed otherwise.

5. A patient who has ulcerative colitis is taken to the emergency department with severe rectal bleeding. Which of the following is the best option for maintaining nutritional status for this patient with ulcerative colitis who must be nil per os (NPO) for an extended period of time?
   1. Nasogastric tube feedings
   2. Percutaneous endoscopic gastrostomy tube feedings
   3. Parenteral nutrition
   4. Intravenous 5% dextrose and water

6. A patient is diagnosed with acute diverticulitis. Which of the following collected data does the nurse recognize may have placed the patient at risk for developing diverticulitis?
   1. A low-fiber diet
   2. Chronic diarrhea
   3. Nonsteroidal anti-inflammatory drug use
   4. Family history of colon cancer

7. Which of the following nursing diagnoses is most appropriate for the nurse to contribute to the plan of care for a patient with symptoms of a bowel obstruction?
   1. *Self-Care Deficit: Feeding* related to nil per os (NPO) status
   2. *Acute Urinary Retention* related to fluid volume depletion
   3. *Risk for Deficient Fluid Volume* related to nausea and vomiting
   4. *Ineffective Coping* related to prolonged hospitalization

8. Which of the following explanations by the nurse to reinforce the patient's preoperative education for a loop ostomy would be correct?
   1. "You will have a stoma in the middle of your abdomen that will constantly drain liquid stool."
   2. "You will have a looped bag system to collect stool from your stoma."
   3. "You will have a loop of bowel on your abdomen, but it will not drain stool."
   4. "You will have a loop of bowel on your abdomen that can be returned to your abdomen after your bowel has healed."

9. Which of the following dietary instructions is most important to include in the plan of care to prevent complications for a patient with an ileostomy?
   1. "Drink adequate fluids to prevent dehydration."
   2. "Avoid fruits and vegetables to prevent diarrhea."
   3. "Avoid milk products to prevent gas."
   4. "Eat plenty of fiber to prevent constipation."

10. A patient is wondering about ileostomy odor and is provided information by the nurse. Which of the following responses by the patient would indicate that teaching has been effective? **Select all that apply.**
    1. "A teaspoon of baking soda in your pouch will absorb all the odor."
    2. "The plastic in the pouch is odor-proof, so there is no odor as long as there is no leak."
    3. "Effluent from an ileostomy can have an odor."
    4. "Changing your pouch and face plate daily will help prevent odor."
    5. "Colostomies are the only ostomy that can smell bad from time to time."

11. The nurse is counseling a patient with frequent anal fissures and a history of constipation. Which of the following patient statements indicates that further teaching is required? **Select all that apply.**
    1. "There isn't much I can do except seek pain relief whenever I have a fissure."
    2. "It is important that I not ignore the urge to have a bowel movement."
    3. "Decreasing the amount of fluid I drink each day will reduce stool frequency and subsequent irritation."
    4. "Opioid analgesics medications are probably needed to help with this condition."
    5. "Sitz baths may provide healing and comfort."
    6. "I should eat a high-fiber diet."

12. The nurse is caring for a patient who has normal saline infusing. The patient suddenly requests assistance to the bedside commode and has bright red liquid stools and reports feeling weak and having visual disturbances. Which actions should the nurse take immediately? **Rank these nursing actions in order of priority.**
    1. Notify health care provider.
    2. Measure output.
    3. Obtain vital signs.
    4. Check patency of intravenous site and infusion.
    5. Assist patient into bed.
    6. Cover with warm blankets.
    7. Identify level of consciousness.
    8. Perform rapid head-to-toe assessment.

13. The nurse is caring for a patient with suspected appendicitis. Mark the area where the pain (a classic symptom of appendicitis) localizes.

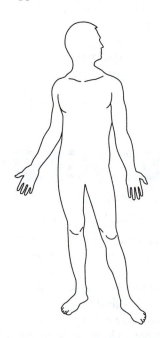

14. The nurse is caring for a patient who has had repair of a right inguinal hernia. Mark the area where the nurse would view the surgical site.

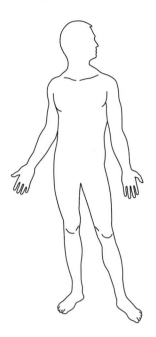

15. The nurse is caring for a patient who has had an ostomy created, which will produce soft to hard formed effluent. Mark the area where the nurse would observe this stoma.

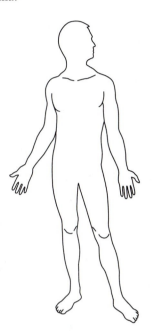

CHAPTER 35
Nursing Care of Patients With Liver, Pancreatic, and Gallbladder Disorders

Name: _____

Date: _____

Course: _____

Instructor: _____

AUDIO CASE STUDY

Listen to the audio case study available on Davis Edge and then answer the following questions.

Kelsey and Cirrhosis

1. What are causes of cirrhosis?

   _____

   _____

   _____

2. What signs of cirrhosis and hepatic encephalopathy (HE), a complication of cirrhosis, is Mr. Guido exhibiting?

   _____

   _____

   _____

   _____

3. What serum lab value is elevated, which contributes to HE?

   _____

   _____

4. What medication is ordered to reduce ammonia levels for Mr. Guido?

   _____

   _____

VOCABULARY

Match the following terms with the appropriate description.

1. _____ Ascites
2. _____ Asterixis
3. _____ Cirrhosis
4. _____ Encephalopathy
5. _____ Fetor hepaticus
6. _____ Hepatorenal syndrome
7. _____ Hepatitis
8. _____ Jaundice
9. _____ Portal hypertension
10. _____ Pancreatectomy
11. _____ Steatorrhea
12. _____ Varices

1. Yellowing of the sclerae and skin from excess bilirubin
2. Removal of all or part of the pancreas
3. Liver flap
4. Fluid in abdominal cavity from decreased albumin level
5. Neurological changes from excess ammonia
6. Weakened, swollen veins
7. Foul breath
8. Increased pressure in the portal circulation
9. Fatty, foul-smelling stools
10. Scarring and hardening of the liver from inflammation
11. Oliguria and sodium retention without kidney defects
12. Inflammation of liver cells

LIVER

Fill in the crossword with terms related to the liver.

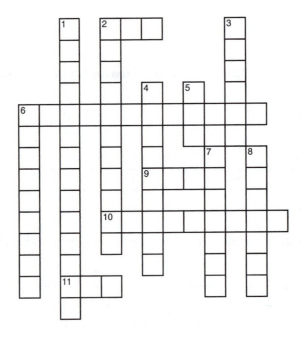

Across

2. Abbreviation for serum hepatitis
6. Visible veins around umbilicus
9. Abbreviation for liver shunt
10. Liver flap
11. Abbreviation for infectious hepatitis

Down

1. Confusion and coma are symptoms
2. This syndrome causes oliguria
3. Abdominal circulation
4. Liver inflammation
5. Abbreviation for location of liver
6. Progressive, irreversible replacement of liver tissue with scar tissue
7. Collection of fluid in abdominal cavity
8. Dilated esophageal veins

GALLBLADDER

Match the following terms with the appropriate description.

1. _____ Cholecystitis
2. _____ Cholesterol
3. _____ Flatulence
4. _____ Murphy sign
5. _____ Bilirubin
6. _____ Cholelithiasis
7. _____ T-tube
8. _____ Choledochoscopy
9. _____ Ultrasound
10. _____ Laparoscopic cholecystectomy

1. Pigment from the breakdown of hemoglobin in red blood cells
2. Classic test done to detect gallstones
3. Use of an endoscope to explore the common bile duct
4. Inflammation of the gallbladder
5. Inability to take a deep breath when fingers are pressed under liver margin
6. Most common substance found in gallstones
7. Intestinal gas expelled via the rectum
8. Gallstones within the gallbladder
9. A surgical drain ensuring bile drains freely from the gallbladder after surgery
10. Removal of the gallbladder through a small abdominal incision

PANCREAS

In the space on the left, write N or A to indicate whether the data collected is normal or abnormal. If the finding is abnormal, indicate the cause for the finding.

1. _____ Serum glucose more than 150 mg
2. _____ Serum amylase more than 500 international unit/L
3. _____ Serum lipase = 15 unit/L
4. _____ Pleural effusion
5. _____ Blood pressure and pulse 15% from patient's baseline

6. _____ Jaundice
7. _____ Presence of Cullen sign
8. _____ Presence of Turner sign
9. _____ Positive Chvostek sign
10. _____ Foul-smelling, fatty stools

CRITICAL THINKING

Read the following case study and answer the questions.

Ms. Bettina Smythe has been diagnosed with hepatic encephalopathy (HE) secondary to cirrhosis. During the admission process, the nurse notes the following findings: abdomen grossly distended, yellow sclerae and skin, multiple bruises, and pitting edema of the lower extremities. The nurse also notes that Ms. Smythe is irritable and that she has difficulty answering questions and appears to doze off frequently during the interview. The nurse observes that Ms. Smythe scratches her arms and legs frequently. Her laboratory data indicate that her serum bilirubin, ammonia, and prothrombin time are elevated and that her serum albumin, total protein, and potassium are below normal.

1. What data support the diagnosis of cirrhosis?

_____

_____

_____

_____

_____

_____

2. What data suggest that Ms. Smythe has HE? What other evidence might the nurse observe?

    _____

    _____

    _____

    _____

    _____

    _____

3. Why is Ms. Smythe exhibiting pitting edema and abdominal distention? _____

    _____

    _____

    _____

    _____

4. What medical treatments can the nurse expect will be ordered for HE?

    _____

    _____

    _____

    Two days after Ms. Smythe is admitted, there is bright red blood in her emesis. Ms. Smythe also reports feeling cold, and her pulse is 115 beats per minute and thready. The nurse calls for help and places Ms. Smythe on her side.

5. What further treatment can be anticipated for Ms. Smythe?

    _____

    _____

    _____

    _____

6. What observations should be made to detect bleeding from lack of clotting factors? _____

    _____

    _____

    _____

    _____

7. What nursing measures can be provided to help Ms. Smythe maintain her fluid balance?

    _____

    _____

    _____

    _____

    _____

8. What should Ms. Smythe be taught about taking acetaminophen (Tylenol)? Why?

    _____

    _____

    _____

REVIEW QUESTIONS—CONTENT REVIEW

Choose the best answer unless directed otherwise.

1. Which of the following precautions will protect the nurse who is caring for the patient with hepatitis B?
   1. Reverse isolation
   2. Standard precautions
   3. Respiratory precautions
   4. Enteric precautions

2. Acute liver failure is most often caused by which of the following?
   1. Antibiotic use
   2. Daily vitamins
   3. Alcohol use
   4. Acetaminophen (Tylenol) overdose

3. Which of the following is a treatment for bleeding esophageal varices? **Select all that apply.**
   1. Variceal ligation (banding)
   2. Octreotide (Sandostatin) intravenously
   3. Soft diet
   4. Clear liquid diet
   5. Transjugular intrahepatic portosystemic shunt

4. A patient with cirrhosis has asterixis and fetor hepaticus and is confused. The nurse recognizes these as symptoms of which complication?
   1. Hepatic encephalopathy
   2. Hepatorenal syndrome
   3. Portal hypertension
   4. Ascites

5. Patients with a history of pancreatitis commonly have a history of which of the following?
   1. High-protein diet
   2. Very-low-fat diet
   3. Excessive alcohol consumption
   4. Excessive intake of vitamin K

REVIEW QUESTIONS—TEST PREPARATION

Choose the best answer unless directed otherwise.

6. The nurse is collecting data for a patient with acute pancreatitis. Which of these descriptions of pain would the nurse associate with acute pancreatitis?
   1. Dull, boring, beginning in the mid-epigastrium and radiating to the back
   2. Knifelike, centered in the left lower quadrant
   3. Burning, focused over the left flank and radiating to the shoulder
   4. Sharp, severe pain that begins in the right upper quadrant

7. A patient with ascites is placed on a low-sodium diet. The nurse knows that diet teaching has been successful if the patient selects which of the following meals?
   1. Cottage cheese and peaches with tomato juice
   2. Frankfurter on a bun with pickle relish and skim milk
   3. Baked chicken, brown rice, and apple juice
   4. Turkey and lettuce sandwich on whole-wheat bread with tomato soup

8. The nurse is collecting data for a patient admitted with possible cholecystitis. Which of the following does the nurse recognize as risk factors for gallbladder disease? **Select all that apply.**
   1. Male gender
   2. Obesity
   3. Multiple pregnancies
   4. Age 40 or older
   5. Fasting
   6. Diabetes mellitus

9. Which of the following instructions should the nurse include in the teaching plan for the patient with portal hypertension? **Select all that apply.**
   1. Cough and deep breathe every 2 hours.
   2. Avoid straining to have a bowel movement.
   3. Avoid heavy lifting
   4. Increase fluid intake.
   5. Take vitamin K supplement.
   6. Consult health care provider before use of aspirin.

10. The nurse provides teaching on prevention of hepatitis. The nurse recognizes the patient requires further instruction if the patient states which of the following? **Select all that apply.**
    1. "I should receive the vaccine for hepatitis A virus."
    2. "I should receive the vaccine for hepatitis B virus."
    3. "I should receive the vaccine for hepatitis C virus."
    4. "I should receive the vaccine for hepatitis D virus."
    5. "Hand washing is important after use of the bathroom."
    6. "I can share my razor."

11. The nurse provides teaching on medications that contain acetaminophen to use cautiously for a patient with cirrhosis. Which of these medications would the patient correctly state should be used cautiously?
    1. Norco
    2. NyQuil
    3. Penicillin
    4. Percocet
    5. Tetracycline
    6. Vicodin

12. The nurse is collecting data on a patient with hepatitis. Which of the following signs or symptoms are a priority for the nurse to report? **Select all that apply.**
    1. Bruising
    2. Fever
    3. Nausea
    4. Malaise
    5. Pruritus

13. The nurse is collecting data on a patient with acute pancreatitis. Mark the area where the nurse would look for the presence of Cullen sign.

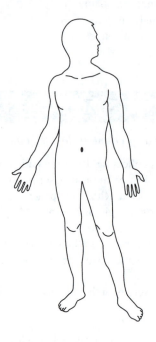

CHAPTER 36

Urinary System Function, Assessment, and Therapeutic Measures

Name: _____	
Date: _____	
Course: _____	
Instructor: _____	

AUDIO CASE STUDY

Listen to the audio case study available on Davis Edge and then answer the following questions.

Adam: Kidney Stones, Cystoscopy, and Pyelogram

1. What type of pain was Adam experiencing with his kidney stone?
   _____
   _____

2. How did the nurse explain renal ultrasound to Adam?
   _____
   _____
   _____
   _____

3. What would have allowed Adam to be discharged prior to having surgery?
   _____
   _____

4. What preoperative care did Adam have?
   _____
   _____
   _____

5. What were the nurses monitoring postoperatively for Adam?

_____

_____

VOCABULARY

Match the term for an abnormality of the urine or urination with the correct description.

1. _____ Hematuria
2. _____ Dysuria
3. _____ Nocturia
4. _____ Oliguria
5. _____ Azotemia
6. _____ Anuria
7. _____ Uremic fetor
8. _____ Calculus

1. Painful urination
2. Decreased urine output (less than 400 mL per 24 hours)
3. Blood in the urine
4. Voiding during the night
5. Stone
6. Absence of urination
7. Excess urea in the blood
8. Urine breath odor

ANATOMY REVIEW

Label the parts of the kidney and nephron.

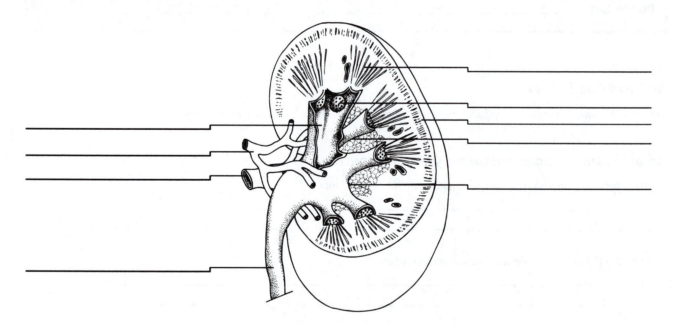

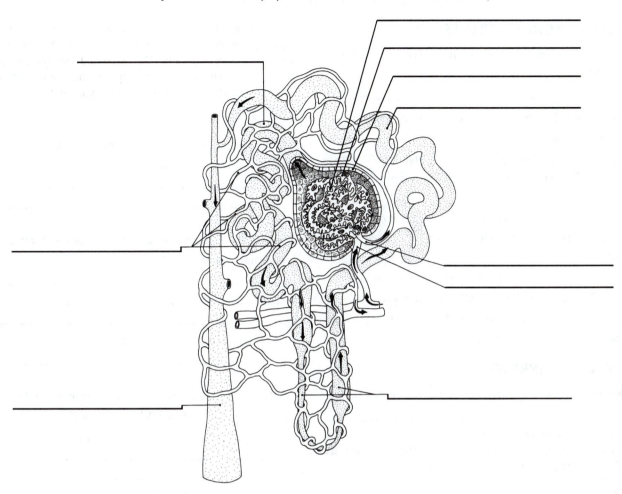

SAMPLE URINALYSIS RESULTS

Review the urinalysis results of the following three patients and determine the most likely cause of the abnormal results.

	Patient A	**Patient B**	**Patient C**
Color	Yellow	Dark amber	Yellow-green
Appearance	Cloudy	Concentrated	Clear
Glucose	Negative	Negative	Negative
Bilirubin	Negative	Negative	2+
Ketones	Small	Negative	Negative
Specific gravity (1.005–1.030)	1.024	1.035	1.025
pH (4.5–8)	6	5.2	5.5
Protein (Less than 20 mg/dL)	100	Negative	Negative
Nitrite	Positive	Negative	Negative
Casts	WBC, RBC	Negative	Negative
White blood cells (0–5 hpf)	400	4	1
Red blood cells (0–5 hpf)	90	2	2
Bacteria (negative)	4+	Negative	Negative

Patient A: _____

_____

Patient B: _____

_____

Patient C: _____

_____

_____

RENAL DIAGNOSTIC TESTS

Label each statement as true or false and correct the false statements.

1. _____ An x-ray of the renal structures after injection of a radiopaque dye into the venous system is called a *renal ultrasound*.

2. _____ A diagnostic test in which sound waves are used to outline the structure of the kidney is a pyelogram.

3. _____ A urine sample that is cultured to determine the kind of bacteria it contains is called a *creatinine clearance urine test*.

4. _____ A diagnostic test in which the inside of the bladder is visualized is called a *cystoscopy*.

5. _____ The radiopaque dye used for diagnostic tests of the renal system is harmless.

CRITICAL THINKING

Read the following case studies and answer the questions.

Mrs. Bohke is a 64-year-old female patient admitted to the hospital with a diagnosis of pneumonia. During her stay, she tells the nurse she has trouble getting to the bathroom in time and often dribbles before she can get there.

1. What type of urinary incontinence does she have?

   _____

   _____

2. What teaching could be done to help her decrease her incontinence?

   _____

   _____

   _____

   _____

Mrs. Simmon is a 79-year-old woman with a fractured hip and a previous cerebrovascular accident (CVA). She has poor vision but is alert mentally. The nurse finds her lying in bed in a puddle of urine, crying. She explains that she was unable to find her call light. The nurse finds it lying on the floor out of her reach.

3. What kind of incontinence did Mrs. Simmon experience?

   _____

   _____

   _____

4. What actions should the nurse take to ensure that this does not happen again?

   _____

   _____

   _____

   _____

   _____

5. When caring for a patient with incontinence, is it helpful to decrease fluid intake? Why or why not?

   _____

   _____

   _____

   _____

REVIEW QUESTIONS—CONTENT REVIEW

Choose the best answer unless otherwise directed.

1. Which of the following is secreted when the blood level of oxygen decreases?
   1. Erythropoietin
   2. Renin
   3. Angiotensin II
   4. Vitamin D

2. Urea is a nitrogenous waste product from the metabolism of which of the following?
   1. Nucleic acids
   2. Amino acids
   3. Muscle tissue
   4. Carbohydrates

3. The kidneys are located behind which of the following structures?
   1. Spinal column
   2. Diaphragm
   3. Peritoneum
   4. Inferior vena cava

4. The renal pyramids make up which kidney structure?
   1. Renal cortex
   2. Renal medulla
   3. Renal pelvis
   4. Renal fascia

5. The process of tubular resorption takes place in which of the following parts of the kidney?
   1. From the glomerulus to the Bowman capsule
   2. From the afferent arteriole to the efferent arteriole
   3. From the peritubular capillaries to the glomerulus
   4. From the renal tubule to the peritubular capillaries

6. Where is urine formed?
   1. Nephrons
   2. Ureters
   3. Urethra
   4. Bladder

7. Which of the following are functions of the kidney? **Select all that apply.**
   1. Maintaining acid–base balance
   2. Removal of waste products
   3. Regulation of the blood volume
   4. Regulation of electrolytes
   5. Removal of carbon dioxide
   6. Production of erythropoietin

REVIEW QUESTIONS—TEST PREPARATION

Choose the best answer unless otherwise directed.

8. When collecting a routine urinalysis specimen on a newly admitted female patient, the nurse should take which of the following actions? **Select all that apply.**
   1. Instruct the patient to wash perineum before collecting the urine specimen.
   2. Ask the patient to void, discard the urine, and then collect the next voiding.
   3. Obtain the last voided urine of the day.
   4. Instruct patient to drink three glasses of water prior to the test.
   5. Instruct the patient to hold the labia open while voiding.

9. A patient's urinalysis results show the following findings: urine: dark amber; bacteria: small; nitrite: negative; specific gravity: 1.035; red blood cells: negative. Which of the following is the best explanation for these results?
   1. Dehydration
   2. Urinary tract infection
   3. Contamination of the specimen from bacteria on the perineum
   4. Contamination from menstruation

10. Which of the following diagnostic test results would the nurse evaluate as being related to renal disease? **Select all that apply.**
    1. Serum hematocrit: 39%
    2. Serum potassium: 4 mEq/L
    3. Serum uric acid: 2 ng/dL
    4. Serum creatinine: 3 mg/dL
    5. Blood urea nitrogen (BUN): 35 mg/dL
    6. Urine specific gravity: 1.020

11. A patient is scheduled for a pyelogram with contrast. When giving care, the nurse should recognize that restriction of which of the following is part of the preparation for a pyelogram?
    1. Salt intake
    2. Fluid intake
    3. Use of tobacco
    4. Physical activities

12. The patient is scheduled for a cystoscopy. Which of the following is the most important nursing care after this kind of surgery?
    1. Measuring urine output.
    2. Monitoring daily weight.
    3. Observing for symptoms of acute kidney injury.
    4. Limiting fluid intake.

13. A patient, age 48, has urge incontinence. When collecting data, the nurse would expect to find which of the following symptoms?
    1. Patient is unable to reach the bathroom in time and ends up urinating in underwear.
    2. Patient is incontinent of small amounts of urine when coughs, sneezes, or bears down.
    3. Patient is incontinent of urine when unable to remove clothing.
    4. Patient is incontinent because unable to tell when needs to urinate and unable to control urination.

14. Which of the following actions should the nurse take to prevent development of a urinary tract infection in a patient who has a urinary catheter inserted? **Select all that apply.**
    1. Limit fluid intake to 1,000 mL per 24 hours to decrease the flow of urine, which can result in increased contamination.
    2. Wash the perineum with an antibacterial soap three times per 24 hours.
    3. Keep catheter securely taped to the patient, preventing back-and-forth motion of the catheter.
    4. Empty the urinary catheter bag only when full.
    5. Prevent contamination of the exit spout when emptying urinary catheter bag.

15. Which of the following actions should the nurse take for a patient who has total urinary incontinence?
    1. Give patient cranberry juice to keep the urine acidic.
    2. Ensure that patient has ready access to the urinal.
    3. Teach patient how to do Kegel exercises to increase perineal tone.
    4. Apply an adult incontinence brief to absorb urine and change when necessary.

16. The nurse is collecting data on a patient with an admission diagnosis of bladder cancer. Which of the following would be expected findings during data collection? **Select all that apply.**
    1. History of smoking
    2. Recent weight gain
    3. Hematuria
    4. Hypertension
    5. Allergy to contrast media
    6. Employed as leather maker

17. A patient with chronic kidney disease has a potassium level of 6 mEq/L The nurse should monitor this patient for which of the following?
    1. Respiratory depression
    2. Cardiac arrhythmias
    3. Hypertension
    4. Urinary retention

18. The nurse is to collect data on a patient's insertion site of a peritoneal dialysis catheter. Mark the area where the nurse would observe the insertion site.

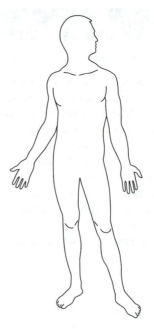

CHAPTER 37

Nursing Care of Patients With Disorders of the Urinary System

Name: _____

Date: _____

Course: _____

Instructor: _____

AUDIO CASE STUDY

Listen to the audio case study available on Davis Edge and then answer the following questions.

Maleka and Kidney Disease

1. What are causes of chronic kidney disease?

   _____

   _____

2. What are causes of acute kidney injury?

   _____

   _____

   _____

3. Before a diagnostic test using contrast media, what actions should be taken to help protect the function of the kidneys?

   _____

   _____

   _____

4. What type of access did Mr. Hopkins have, and how was it monitored?

   _____

   _____

   _____

VOCABULARY

Fill in the blank with the correct term.

1. _____ is inflammation of the urethra.
2. _____ is inflammation of the bladder.
3. _____ is inflammation of the kidney.
4. Surgical repair of the urethra is called _____.
5. Sepsis caused by a severe urinary infection is called _____.
6. A percutaneous _____ is a small surgical incision made in the skin to allow insertion of a nephroscope into the kidney to remove a stone.
7. Unrelieved obstruction of the urinary tract can lead to _____.
8. A _____ tube may be inserted directly into the kidney pelvis to drain urine.
9. Surgical removal of a kidney is called a _____.
10. Thickening and hardening of the renal blood vessels is called _____.

URINARY TRACT INFECTIONS

Answer the following questions.

1. What is the usual cause of urinary tract infections (UTIs) in women?

   _____
   _____
   _____

2. What is the usual cause of UTIs in men?

   _____
   _____
   _____

3. What advice regarding fluids should be given to patients who are susceptible to UTIs?

   _____
   _____
   _____

4. What is the single most important thing a patient with a history of UTIs should be taught?

   _____
   _____

5. What are UTI signs and symptoms found in the older adult?

   _____
   _____

6. Compare cystitis (bladder infection) with pyelonephritis (kidney infection) by filling out the following table.

Things to Compare	Cystitis	Pyelonephritis
Symptoms	_____	_____
	_____	_____
	_____	_____
	_____	_____
	_____	_____
	_____	_____
	_____	_____
	_____	_____
	_____	_____
Urinalysis Results	_____	_____
	_____	_____
	_____	_____
	_____	_____
Prognosis	_____	_____
	_____	_____
	_____	_____
	_____	_____

URINARY TRACT OBSTRUCTIONS

Answer the following questions.

1. What is the most common symptom of cancer of the bladder?

   _____

   _____

2. What is the most common risk factor for cancer of the bladder?

   _____

   _____

3. What is the most common symptom of cancer of the kidney?

   _____

   _____

4. What does urine look like when a patient has an ileal conduit?

   _____

   _____

5. What nursing care should be provided for a patient with an ileal conduit?

   _____

   _____

   _____

   _____

   _____

6. What is the most important care that should be provided for a patient with a kidney stone?

   _____

   _____

7. What teaching should be done for the patient to prevent further stone formation if the stone is composed of calcium oxalate? Uric acid?

   _____

   _____

   _____

   _____

CRITICAL THINKING

Read the following case study and answer the questions.

Mrs. Zins is a 27-year-old woman who has had type 1 diabetes mellitus for more than 20 years. Recently, she has begun having incidents of hypoglycemia, she is edematous, and her blood pressure has elevated. She is admitted to the hospital for diagnosis and treatment of probable chronic kidney disease (CKD).

History: Subjective Data

- States that she has been exhausted lately and her skin is itchy
- States that she has been very irritable and her husband says she is difficult to live with

Physical: Objective Data

- Blood pressure 194/104 mm Hg, pulse 98 beats per minute, respiration 22 per minute, temperature 98.4°F (36.9°C)
- Jugular vein distention present at 45 degrees
- Generalized edema throughout body, including periorbital edema
- Pitting edema of feet and ankles
- Weight gain of 20 pounds in 2 months
- Skin very dry, flaky

Diagnostic Tests

- Fasting blood sugar: 56 mg/100 L
- Serum sodium: 145 mEq/L
- Serum creatinine: 5.4 mg/100 L
- Serum potassium: 5.9 mEq/L
- Uric acid: 8.2 ng/dL
- Hemoglobin (Hgb): 7.2 g/100 mL
- Hematocrit (Hct): 22%

1. Mrs. Zins has been having incidents of hypoglycemia. Why is this happening? _____

   _____

   _____

   _____

2. With Mrs. Zins's present blood sugar of 56, what kind of juice should the nurse give her? _____

   _____

   _____

3. How does diabetes cause CKD? _____

_____

_____

_____

4. Is there anything Mrs. Zins could have done to decrease the possibility of developing CKD? _____

_____

5. Identify two nursing diagnoses that would be appropriate for Mrs. Zins based on her collected data. _____

_____

_____

_____

6. What diagnostic test was most indicative of CKD for Mrs. Zins? _____

_____

7. Why is Mrs. Zins anemic? _____

_____

_____

_____

8. What would be the three most important areas for nursing data collection for Mrs. Zins related to CKD?

_____

_____

_____

9. What kind of diet will Mrs. Zins most likely receive?

_____

_____

_____

_____

_____

CHRONIC KIDNEY DISEASE

Fill in the signs and symptoms of chronic kidney disease under the body systems on the figure that follows.

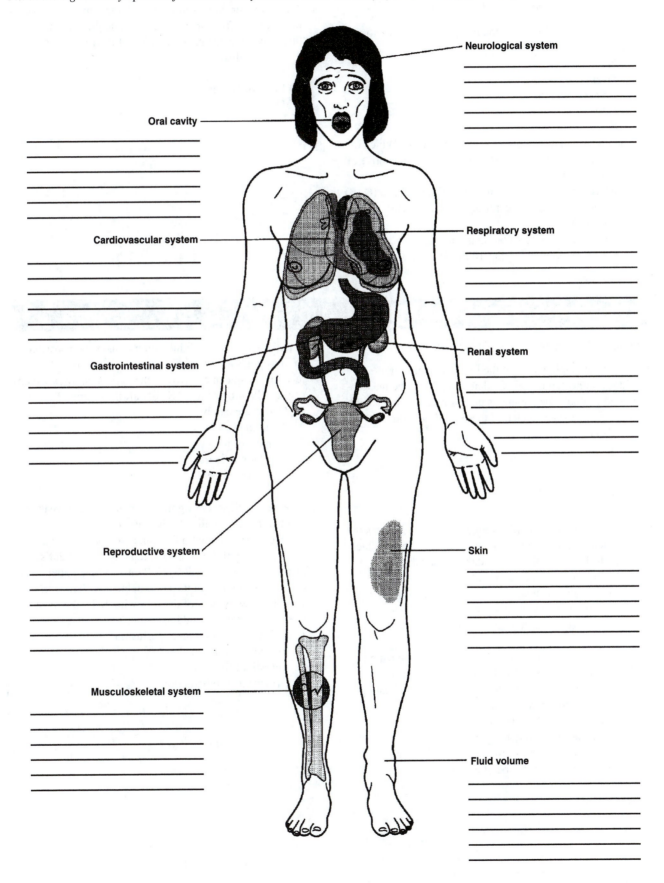

REVIEW QUESTIONS—CONTENT REVIEW

Choose the best answer unless directed otherwise.

1. Which of the following is the most common symptom of cancer of the bladder?
   1. Nocturia
   2. Dysuria
   3. Urinary retention
   4. Hematuria

2. The nurse reviews a patient's diagnostic tests. Which of the patient's diagnostic tests results is most indicative of acute kidney injury?
   1. Blood urea nitrogen: 80 mg/100 mL (8–25 mg/100 L)
   2. 24-hour creatinine clearance: 5 mL/min (100 mL/min)
   3. Uric acid: 8 ng/dL (2.5–5.5 ng/dL)
   4. Serum creatinine: 1.7 mg/100 L (0.5–1.5 mg/100 L)

3. A patient's urinalysis indicates a large amount of protein in the urine. The nurse recognizes that this finding most likely indicates damage to which of the following?
   1. Glomerulus
   2. Renal pelvis
   3. Loop of Henle
   4. Ureter

REVIEW QUESTIONS—TEST PREPARATION

Choose the best answer unless directed otherwise.

4. The nurse taught a patient the foods to avoid for a kidney stone composed of calcium oxalate. The nurse would evaluate the patient as understanding the teaching if the patient states which of these foods should be avoided?
   1. Bread
   2. Beer
   3. Beef
   4. Beans

5. Following a urostomy (ileal conduit), the nurse notes the presence of mucus in the patient's urostomy bag. Which of the following actions should the nurse take?
   1. Notify the health care provider.
   2. Collect a urine specimen for culture and sensitivity.
   3. Measure the specific gravity of the urine.
   4. Recognize this as a normal occurrence.

6. The nurse is collecting data for a postoperative patient. Which of the following findings would the nurse recognize as being the most significant sign indicating acute kidney injury has occurred?
   1. A decrease in blood pressure
   2. An elevation in body temperature
   3. A decrease in urine output
   4. An increase in urine specific gravity

7. A patient with acute kidney injury has been instructed to limit potassium intake. The nurse recognizes that teaching has been effective if the patient chooses which of the following snacks? **Select all that apply.**
   1. Chocolate candy
   2. An orange
   3. Grapefruit juice
   4. A gelatin dessert
   5. Cranberry juice

8. A patient with severe right flank pain, general weakness, and fever is hospitalized. The patient has a history of recurrent urinary tract infection, and renal calculi are suspected. On the second hospital day, the patient's urine output drops to 300 mL/24 hr, and the patient has distention and pain in the suprapubic area. The nurse would suspect which of the following to be the most likely cause for this sudden change?
   1. Sudden decreased renal perfusion
   2. Inadequate fluid intake
   3. Interstitial fluid shift
   4. Urinary tract obstruction

9. The nurse teaches a patient how to obtain a midstream urine specimen for culture and sensitivity. The nurse would evaluate the patient as understanding the teaching if the patient states which of these?
   1. "I will collect the second-voided specimen in the morning."
   2. "The specimen should be collected early in the morning."
   3. "I should begin voiding, collect the specimen, and then finish voiding in the toilet."
   4. "A 24-hour urine specimen is needed; the first void should be discarded and then the 24-hour timing begun."

10. A patient is admitted with chronic kidney disease. The patient, who has a potassium level of 6.4 mEq/L, is placed on a cardiac monitor and given sodium polystyrene sulfonate (kayexalate) by retention enema. Which of the following is the most significant symptom that should be monitored during data collection?
    1. Diarrhea
    2. Irregular heart rhythm
    3. Increased blood pressure
    4. Increased respiratory rate

11. The nursing diagnosis of *Excess Fluid Volume* is made for a patient with chronic kidney disease. Which of the following data is most important for the nurse to collect for this patient based on the nursing diagnosis?
    1. Intake and output
    2. Vital signs
    3. Daily weight
    4. Skin turgor

12. A patient with newly diagnosed chronic kidney disease has elevated serum sodium, potassium, and creatinine levels. The patient's breakfast is delivered and includes a glass of orange juice. Which of the following actions should the nurse take?
    1. Encourage the patient to drink the orange juice for vitamin C to help fight the infection.
    2. Remove the orange juice from the tray because it is high in potassium.
    3. Give the patient a smaller glass of orange juice to limit fluids.
    4. Check the type of diet the patient has prescribed to determine restrictions.

13. A patient is scheduled for surgery to create an arteriovenous fistula for dialysis. The patient asks why it needs to be done. Which of the following is the best explanation by the nurse on the advantages of a fistula over a two-tailed subclavian catheter? **Select all that apply.**
    1. "There is greater blood flow with a fistula."
    2. "There is less risk of clotting with the fistula."
    3. "It is easier to access the fistula than the two-tailed subclavian."
    4. "The fistula is less likely to be damaged by trauma."
    5. "The fistula has less risk of infection."

14. After hemodialysis, which of the following nursing interventions are a priority for the nurse to carry out? **Select all that apply.**
    1. Document stool output.
    2. Weigh the patient.
    3. Check for jugular vein distention.
    4. Obtain vital signs.
    5. Allow patient to rest.
    6. Provide meal.

15. The patient has a permanent peritoneal catheter inserted and is begun on continuous ambulatory peritoneal dialysis. The patient asks how this dialysis works. Which of the following would be the best explanation by the nurse of how this type of dialysis works?
    1. "The peritoneum allows solutes in the dialysate to pass into the intravascular system."
    2. "The peritoneum acts as a semipermeable membrane through which solutes move by diffusion and osmosis."
    3. "The presence of excess metabolites causes increased permeability of the peritoneum and allows excess fluid to drain."
    4. "The peritoneum permits diffusion of metabolites from the intravascular to the interstitial space."

16. A patient undergoing dialysis has a severe cerebrovascular accident and is now semicomatose. His family decides, according to the patient's advance directive, that dialysis should be stopped. He is sent home with his daughter for hospice. As part of discharge planning, his daughter should be taught to expect which of the following signs and symptoms of untreated end-stage renal failure? **Select all that apply.**
    1. Polyuria
    2. Dehydration
    3. Edema
    4. Possible convulsions
    5. Urea skin crystals
    6. Pruritis

17. A patient is admitted who was involved in a motor vehicle accident resulting in trauma to the abdomen and back. The patient has a ruptured spleen and probable trauma to the kidneys. The nurse should monitor for which of the following changes related to the patient's urinary output?
    1. Dysuria
    2. Pyuria
    3. Polyuria
    4. Hematuria

18. A patient is admitted with symptoms of recent weight gain, pitting edema of the feet, jugular vein distention, and lung crackles. Which of the following nursing diagnoses is most appropriate for this patient's plan of care?
    1. *Risk for Deficient Fluid Volume*
    2. *Excess Fluid Volume*
    3. *Imbalanced Nutrition: Less Than Body Requirements*
    4. *Powerlessness*

19. A patient has renal failure and is oliguric. It would be best for the nurse to determine this patient's fluid balance by monitoring which of the following?
    1. Blood pressure
    2. Fluid intake
    3. Hemoglobin
    4. Weight gain

20. Which of the following are interventions the nurse should implement when caring for a patient who has a left arm arteriovenous fistula? **Select all that apply.**
    1. Check fistula bruit and thrill.
    2. Keep fistula covered with a dry sterile dressing.
    3. Keep the fistula dry.
    4. Take blood pressure on right arm.
    5. Obtain lab draws on left arm.
    6. Insert intravenous line for medications in right arm.

CHAPTER 38
Endocrine System Function and Assessment

Name: _____
Date: _____
Course: _____
Instructor: _____

AUDIO CASE STUDY

Listen to the audio case study available on Davis Edge and then answer the following questions.

NANCY HAS HYPERTHYROIDISM

1. What symptoms of hyperthyroidism did Nancy experience?

_____

_____

_____

_____

_____

2. Why was her thyroid-stimulating hormone (TSH) level below normal?

_____

_____

_____

_____

_____

3. What precautions did she have to take after her thyroid scan?

_____

_____

_____

_____

_____

VOCABULARY

Complete the following sentences with the appropriate words.

1. Glucose is converted to _____ for storage.

2. High blood glucose is called _____.

3. Emotional tone is called _____.

4. Bulging eyes, called _____, is a symptom of hyperthyroidism.

5. Hormone secretion is regulated through a _____ system.

HORMONES

Match each hormone with its function. Use each number only once.

1. _____ Antidiuretic hormone (ADH)

2. _____ Oxytocin

3. _____ Thyroid-stimulating hormone (TSH)

4. _____ Adrenocorticotropic hormone

5. _____ Growth hormone (GH)

6. _____ Prolactin

7. _____ Follicle-stimulating hormone (FSH)

8. _____ Luteinizing hormone (LH)

9. _____ Thyroxine

10. _____ Calcitonin

11. _____ Parathyroid hormone

12. _____ Epinephrine

13. _____ Norepinephrine

14. _____ Cortisol

15. _____ Aldosterone

16. _____ Insulin

17. _____ Glucagon

1. Stimulates growth and secretions of the thyroid gland

2. Increases glucose uptake by cells and glycogen storage in the liver

3. Decreases the resorption of calcium from bones; lowers blood calcium level

4. Increases the use of fats and amino acids for energy and has an anti-inflammatory effect

5. Stimulates mitosis and protein synthesis

6. Increases heart rate and force of contraction

7. Causes vasoconstriction throughout the body

8. Increases secretion of cortisol by the adrenal cortex

9. Increases energy production for a normal metabolic rate

10. Directly increases water reabsorption by the kidneys

11. In men, stimulates secretion of testosterone

12. Increases the conversion of glycogen to glucose in the liver between meals

13. Initiates milk production in the mammary glands

14. Increases the resorption of calcium from bones; raises blood calcium level

15. Increases the reabsorption of sodium by the kidneys

16. In women, initiates development of ova in ovaries

17. Causes contraction of the myometrium during labor

ENDOCRINE GLANDS AND HORMONES

Label the figure with the glands of the endocrine system. List the hormone(s) secreted by each gland.

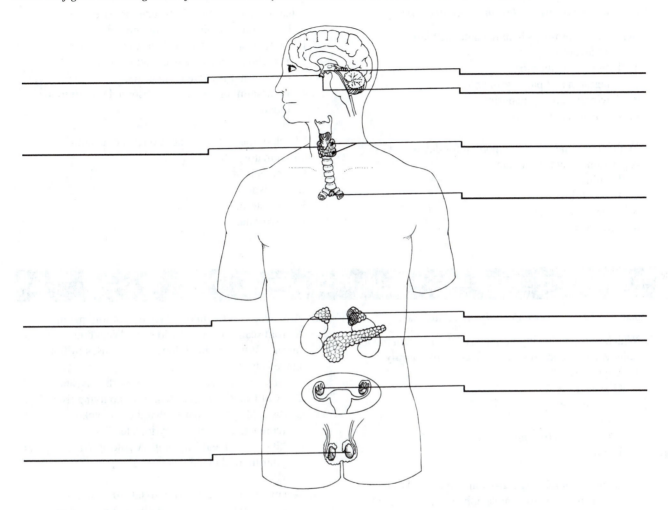

REVIEW QUESTIONS—CONTENT REVIEW

Choose the best answer unless directed otherwise.

1. Which two hormones help regulate the blood calcium level?
   1. Insulin and glucagon
   2. Calcitonin and parathyroid hormone
   3. Thyroxine and epinephrine
   4. Cortisol and aldosterone

2. Which hormone is most important for day-to-day regulation of metabolic rate?
   1. Insulin
   2. Epinephrine
   3. Growth hormone
   4. Thyroxine

3. What happens when aldosterone increases the reabsorption of sodium ions by the kidneys?
   1. Water is also reabsorbed back into the blood.
   2. Bicarbonate ions are excreted in urine.
   3. More water is excreted in urine.
   4. Potassium ions are also reabsorbed back into the blood.

4. Which of the following hormones has an anti-inflammatory effect?
   1. Epinephrine
   2. Cortisol
   3. Aldosterone
   4. Thyroxine

REVIEW QUESTIONS—TEST PREPARATION

Choose the best answer unless directed otherwise.

5. Which of the following hormones help maintain blood volume and blood pressure? **Select all that apply.**
   1. Thyroxine
   2. Glucagon
   3. Aldosterone
   4. Cortisol
   5. Antidiuretic hormone
   6. Insulin

6. A patient is completing a 24-hour urine test. What should the nurse do to complete the test at the end of the 24 hours?
   1. Have the patient void exactly 24 hours after the test was begun and discard the specimen.
   2. Save the last specimen and send it in a separate container.
   3. Have the patient void exactly 24 hours after the test was begun and add this urine to the remainder of the specimen.
   4. Send only the specimen voided at 24 hours.

7. A female patient is admitted to the hospital with hyperthyroidism. What related assessment should the nurse perform?
   1. Check the patient's heart rate.
   2. Palpate the thyroid gland for enlargement.
   3. Do a capillary blood glucose level.
   4. Observe for a "buffalo hump" on the patient's back.

8. A patient asks the nurse, "My doctor told me my thyroid scan showed a 'cold spot.' What does that mean?" Which of the following responses by the nurse is best?
   1. "That means you have cancer of the thyroid gland."
   2. "Cold spots are areas that have no living tissue."
   3. "A cold spot is an area that did not pick up the radioactive material they injected."
   4. "It doesn't mean anything. A cold spot is just part of your thyroid gland."

9. A patient has a prescription to take 0.15 mg of synthetic thyroid hormone daily. The pill is dispensed in micrograms (mcg). How many mcg should the patient take? _____ mcg

10. How do incretin hormones glucagon-like peptide (GLP-1) and gastric inhibitory polypeptide (GIP) help regulate blood sugar after an individual has ingested food? **Select all that apply.**
    1. Increase stimulation of gastric enzymes
    2. Increase insulin secretion from the pancreas
    3. Decrease cellular uptake of glucose
    4. Decrease glucagon secretion from the pancreas
    5. Increase glucose clearance by the kidneys

CHAPTER 39
Nursing Care of Patients With Endocrine Disorders

Name:	
Date:	
Course:	
Instructor:	

AUDIO CASE STUDY

Listen to the audio case study available on Davis Edge and then answer the following questions.

Alice and Cushing Syndrome

1. What was the cause of Alice's Cushing syndrome?

_____

_____

_____

_____

2. What are three or four symptoms of Cushing syndrome?

_____

_____

_____

_____

3. Why did Alice need her blood glucose checked?

_____

_____

_____

_____

4. Are there ways to reduce symptoms of Cushing syndrome?

_____

_____

_____

_____

VOCABULARY

Use the following terms to fill in the blanks.

Amenorrhea	Nocturia
Ectopic	Polydipsia
Euthyroid	Polyuria
Goitrogen	Tetany
Myxedema	Pheochromocytoma

1. A normally functioning thyroid gland produces a _____ state.

2. A food or medication that can cause enlargement of the thyroid gland is called a

   _____.

3. Excessive thirst is called _____.

4. Excessive urination is called _____.

5. A _____ is a tumor of the adrenal medulla.

6. Muscle spasms and tingling around the mouth are symptoms of _____.

7. Untreated hypothyroidism can lead to _____ coma.

8. _____ is the word for getting up to void during the night.

9. Absence of menses is called _____.

10. Sometimes hormones are produced outside the endocrine gland in a/an _____
    site.

HORMONES

Match each disorder to the related hormone imbalance and major signs and symptoms.

Disorder	Hormone Problem	Major Signs and Symptoms
_____ A. Diabetes insipidus	1. Antidiuretic hormone (ADH) deficiency	a. Polyuria
_____ B. Syndrome of inappropriate antidiuretic hormone (SIADH)	2. Growth hormone (GH) deficiency	b. Growing hands and feet
_____ C. Cushing syndrome	3. High serum calcium	c. Moon face
_____ D. Addison's disease	4. ADH excess	d. Unstable hypertension
_____ E. Graves' disease	5. Steroid excess	e. Tetany
_____ F. Hypothyroidism	6. Deficient steroids	f. Muscle weakness, brittle bones
_____ G. Pheochromocytoma	7. Epinephrine excess	g. Failure to grow and develop
_____ H. Hyperparathyroidism	8. GH excess	h. Water retention
_____ I. Short stature	9. Low triiodothyronine (T_3) and thyroxine (T_4)	i. Weight gain and fatigue
_____ J. Acromegaly	10. Low serum calcium	j. Exophthalmos
_____ K. Hypoparathyroidism	11. High T_3 and T_4	k. Hypotension

CRITICAL THINKING

Read the following case studies and answer the questions.

Mr. Samuels is diagnosed with SIADH related to lung cancer. He enters the hospital for treatment of symptoms.

1. What (fluid-related) nursing diagnosis would be most appropriate for Mr. Samuels?

   _____

   _____

2. How will you monitor Mr. Samuels's fluid balance?

   _____

   _____

   _____

3. Why is Mr. Samuels at risk for seizures?

   _____

   _____

   _____

4. How will you reduce his risk for injury from seizures?

   _____

   _____

5. What do you expect to observe when assessing Mr. Samuels's urine?

   _____

   _____

6. What urine characteristics do you expect to observe after treatment has begun?

   _____

   _____

Mrs. Jorgensen is hospitalized following a motor vehicle accident in which she sustained a head injury. She develops diabetes insipidus (DI).

7. Why does head injury place Mrs. Jorgensen at risk for DI?

   _____

   _____

   _____

8. What symptoms do DI and diabetes mellitus (DM) have in common?

   _____

   _____

9. Will Mrs. Jorgensen's urine specific gravity be high or low? Why

   _____

   _____

10. Will Mrs. Jorgensen's serum osmolality be high or low? Why?

    _____

    _____

11. For which (body fluid-related) nursing diagnosis is Mrs. Jorgensen at risk?

    _____

    _____

12. Mrs. Jorgensen begins treatment with DDAVP (desmopressin acetate tablets). What signs of overdose should Mrs. Jorgensen be aware of?

    _____

    _____

THYROID DISORDERS

Label each symptom with an R if it suggests hyperthyroidism or an O if it suggests hypothyroidism.

1. _____ Bradycardia
2. _____ Lethargy
3. _____ Restlessness
4. _____ Frequent stools
5. _____ Hypercholesterolemia
6. _____ Dry hair
7. _____ Tremor
8. _____ Insomnia
9. _____ Mental dullness, confusion
10. _____ Warm, diaphoretic skin
11. _____ Weight loss
12. _____ Decreased appetite

REVIEW QUESTIONS—CONTENT REVIEW

Choose the best answer unless directed otherwise.

1. Following surgery for thyroidectomy, the nurse watches carefully for which of the following signs and symptoms of tetany?
   1. Numb fingers, muscle cramps
   2. Weakness, muscle fatigue
   3. Hallucinations, delusions
   4. Dyspnea and tachycardia

2. What assessment findings should the nurse monitor to detect the onset of thyrotoxicosis in a patient with hyperthyroidism?
   1. Peripheral pulses
   2. Serum sodium
   3. Vital signs
   4. Incision site

3. Which of the following dietary recommendations will reduce the risk of kidney stones in the patient with hyperparathyroidism?
   1. Increase fluids
   2. Increase citrus fruits
   3. Limit meat products
   4. Limit bread products

4. An excess of which hormone is responsible for acromegaly?
   1. Thyroid-stimulating hormone
   2. Insulin
   3. Adrenocorticotropic hormone
   4. Growth hormone

5. Which of the following nursing diagnoses is most appropriate for the patient admitted in addisonian crisis?
   1. *Imbalanced Nutrition: More Than Body Requirements*
   2. *Deficient Fluid Volume*
   3. *Disturbed Body Image*
   4. *Acute Pain*

REVIEW QUESTIONS—TEST PREPARATION

Choose the best answer unless directed otherwise.

6. A 42-year-old patient enters an outpatient clinic with symptoms of weight gain and fatigue. Laboratory studies are done, and a diagnosis of primary hypothyroidism is made. The patient asks why the thyroid-stimulating hormone level is elevated. Which of the following is the best response by the nurse?
   1. "The thyroid makes more thyroid-stimulating hormone to take the place of the deficient triiodothyronine (T_3) and thyroxine (T_4)."
   2. "The thyroid-stimulating hormone tries to directly raise the metabolic rate when there is not enough triiodothyronine (T_3) and thyroxine (T_4)."
   3. "The pituitary makes more thyroid-stimulating hormone to try to stimulate the underactive thyroid."
   4. "The extra fat cells from your weight gain make excess thyroid-stimulating hormone."

7. Which of the following nursing diagnoses would be most appropriate for a patient with fatigue related to hypothyroidism?
   1. *Imbalanced Nutrition: More Than Body Requirements* related to excessive food intake
   2. *Impaired Gas Exchange* related to weight gain
   3. *Activity Intolerance* related to fatigue
   4. *Ineffective Coping* related to depression

8. A patient with hypothyroidism is started on levothyroxine (Synthroid). Which of the following statements shows that the patient understands teaching related to the new medication?
   1. "I know I should call my doctor if my heart races."
   2. "I understand that I may develop a moon-shaped face."
   3. "The sleepiness I experience when I start this medication will subside within 2 weeks."
   4. "I'll have to watch my diet to avoid further weight gain while on this medication."

9. A 26-year-old patient is hospitalized for radioactive iodine treatment for hyperthyroidism. Which of the following precautions by the nurse is appropriate?
   1. Talk with the patient only over the intercom system.
   2. Wear gloves when emptying the bedside commode.
   3. Maintain reverse isolation for 3 months.
   4. No precautions are necessary because the dose is so small.

10. The nurse needs to accomplish all the following interventions for a patient who is 24 hours post-thyroidectomy. Place the interventions in the correct order in which they should be completed.
    1. Check the surgical site dressing for signs of bleeding.
    2. Verify that the airway is patent.
    3. Assess vital signs.
    4. Administer an analgesic for postoperative pain.
    5. Teach the patient about levothyroxine (Synthroid) use after discharge.
    6. Assist with range of motion exercises of the neck.

11. The nurse develops the nursing diagnosis of *Acute Pain* related to bone demineralization for a patient with hyperparathyroidism. Which of the following goals is most appropriate?
    1. Serum calcium level will be less than 20 mg/dL.
    2. Patient will state correct dietary restrictions.
    3. Patient will perform activities of daily living without injury.
    4. Patient will verbalize acceptable pain level.

12. A patient enters a clinic with possible Cushing syndrome. Which of the following physical examination findings support this diagnosis?
    1. Weight loss, pale skin
    2. Buffalo hump, easy bruising
    3. Nausea, vomiting
    4. Polyuria, polydipsia

13. Which data is most important for the nurse to monitor in a patient with a pheochromocytoma?
    1. Vital signs
    2. Daily weights
    3. Peripheral pulses
    4. Bowel sounds

CHAPTER 40

Nursing Care of Patients With Disorders of the Endocrine Pancreas

Name: _____	
Date: _____	
Course: _____	
Instructor: _____	

AUDIO CASE STUDY

Mr. Flint Has Diabetes

Listen to the audio case study available on Davis Edge and then answer the following questions.

1. What risk factors led to the wound on Mr. Flint's foot?

   _____

   _____

2. Why did he need to use crutches to walk?

   _____

   _____

3. What fasting blood glucose level is diagnostic for diabetes?

   _____

   _____

4. What type of diabetes do you think Mr. Flint has? Why?

   _____

   _____

   _____

5. What are three symptoms of hyperglycemia?

   _____

   _____

   _____

6. What are three symptoms of hypoglycemia?

_____

_____

_____

VOCABULARY

Fill in the blanks.

1. Glucose in the urine is called _____.

2. _____ is too much sugar in the blood.

3. _____ is too little sugar in the blood.

4. Deep, sighing respirations from diabetic acidosis are called _____ respirations.

5. Excessive hunger is called _____.

6. Excessive thirst is called _____.

7. The term used to document getting up to urinate at night is _____.

8. The time when insulin is working its hardest after injection is called its _____ action time.

9. The length of time insulin works is called its _____.

10. The Diabetes Control and Complications Trial (DCCT) found that individuals who maintain _____ control of their diabetes will have fewer long-term complications.

HYPOGLYCEMIA AND HYPERGLYCEMIA

Place an R in front of each symptom of hyperglycemia and an O in front of each symptom of hypoglycemia.

1. _____ Tremor

2. _____ Polydipsia

3. _____ Polyuria

4. _____ Lethargy

5. _____ Irritability

6. _____ Fruity breath

7. _____ Sweating

8. _____ Blurred vision

COMPLICATIONS OF DIABETES

Match the complication with its signs and symptoms.

1. _____ Retinopathy

2. _____ Neuropathy

3. _____ Hyperosmolar hyperglycemic state

4. _____ Diabetic ketoacidosis (DKA)

5. _____ Nephropathy

6. _____ Gastroparesis

7. _____ Infection

1. Ketones in the blood and urine

2. Burning pain in legs and feet

3. Fever

4. Lethargy, extreme thirst

5. Impaired vision

6. Food intolerance

7. Microalbuminuria

CRITICAL THINKING

Read the following case study and answer the questions.

Jennie is a 56-year-old overweight woman admitted to your medical unit with cellulitis of the left leg. She has a long history of diabetes mellitus; her blood sugar level is 436. She tells you that she takes insulin glargine (Lantus) 18 units every bedtime and insulin lispro (Humalog) 12 units with each meal. She also takes metformin (Glucophage) twice a day.

1. Jennie tells you that her health care provider wants her to keep her blood sugar level between 100 and 150 mg/dL. You know that a normal blood sugar level is 70 to 100. Why the discrepancy?

   _____

   _____

   _____

   _____

   _____

   _____

2. When you enter Jennie's room to check her 1600 vital signs, she says she has a headache. By the time you finish taking her blood pressure, she has developed a cold sweat. What is happening? What should you do?

   _____

   _____

   _____

   _____

   _____

3. At 1700, you check Jennie's blood sugar level and find that it is 80 mg/dL. What is your next step?

   _____

   _____

   _____

   _____

4. List three things that may have caused Jennie's blood sugar level to drop.

   _____

   _____

   _____

   _____

5. You explain to Jennie the importance of eating three meals a day on a regular schedule. She asks why. How do you explain this to her?

   _____

   _____

   _____

   _____

6. Jennie is discharged and follows her diet, exercise, and insulin regimen carefully. She even loses 50 lb. One year after her first admission, she is brought into the emergency department with a blood sugar level of 32. Why has her blood sugar level dropped?

_____

_____

_____

_____

7. What are two ways that metformin works?

_____

_____

_____

8. Does Jennie have type 1 or type 2 diabetes? How do you know?

_____

_____

_____

_____

_____

REVIEW QUESTIONS—CONTENT REVIEW

Choose the best answer unless directed otherwise.

1. Which of the following is an acceptable premeal blood sugar range for most patients with diabetes?
   1. 46 to 98 mg/dL
   2. 80 to 130 mg/dL
   3. 180 to 250 mg/dL
   4. 350 to 600 mg/dL

2. Before giving insulin, the nurse always checks which test result?
   1. Recent potassium level
   2. Blood glucose level
   3. Urine ketones
   4. White blood cell count

3. At what point after injection does the peak action of insulin lispro (Humalog) occur?
   1. 30 to 90 minutes
   2. 2 to 3 hours
   3. 4 to 5 hours
   4. 8 to 12 hours

4. Which of the following are symptoms of hypoglycemia?
   1. Nausea and vomiting
   2. Glycosuria
   3. Cold sweat and tremor
   4. Polyuria and polydipsia

5. In addition to stimulating insulin production, glyburide (Micronase) has which of the following effects?
   1. Stimulates gluconeogenesis
   2. Promotes fat breakdown
   3. Increases tissue sensitivity to insulin
   4. Enhances appetite

REVIEW QUESTIONS—TEST PREPARATION

Choose the best answer unless directed otherwise.

6. A 26-year-old patient is admitted to the hospital with a new diagnosis of diabetes, a blood glucose level of 680 mg/dL, and ketones in the blood and urine. Which type of diabetes should the nurse suspect?
   1. Type 1
   2. Type 2
   3. Prediabetes
   4. Gestational

7. A patient with diabetes forgot to take a daily dose of glyburide (Micronase). For which of the following symptoms should the nurse be vigilant?
   1. Cold, clammy sweat
   2. Tachycardia, nervousness, hunger
   3. Chest pain, shortness of breath
   4. Fatigue, thirst, blurred vision

8. By which routes can insulin be administered? **Select all that apply.**
   1. Oral
   2. Topical
   3. Intravenous
   4. Subcutaneous
   5. Intramuscular

9. A nurse is preparing a patient with diabetes for a radiological study involving contrast dye. Which of the patient's morning medications should the nurse question?
   1. Sitagliptin (Januvia)
   2. Metformin (Glucophage)
   3. Aspirin (Ecotrin)
   4. Simvastatin (Zocor)

10. A patient with newly diagnosed diabetes asks the nurse what to take for low blood sugar. Which of the following would be most appropriate for the nurse to suggest?
    1. Raisins
    2. Cheese
    3. Acetaminophen (Tylenol)
    4. Beef jerky

11. The nurse recognizes that teaching is effective if a patient with diabetes knows to use subcutaneous glucagon for an emergency episode of which of the following conditions?
    1. Hyperglycemia
    2. Ketonuria
    3. Diabetic ketoacidosis
    4. Hypoglycemia

12. A patient on a carbohydrate counting meal plan receives a breakfast tray and does not care for the oatmeal. Which of the following foods can the nurse substitute for a half cup of oatmeal?
    1. Two eggs
    2. Two strips of bacon
    3. 1 oz of cheese
    4. A slice of wheat toast

13. Mark the eight areas on the body where subcutaneous insulin injections can be administered.

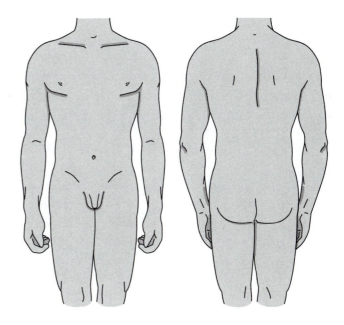

CHAPTER 41

Genitourinary and Reproductive System Function and Assessment

Name: _____

Date: _____

Course: _____

Instructor: _____

AUDIO CASE STUDY

Listen to the audio case study available on Davis Edge and then answer the following questions.

Emma and Lily—Women's Health

1. What measures of comfort can you provide for a woman undergoing a pelvic examination and Pap smear?

   _____

   _____

   _____

   _____

2. What did Emma teach Lily about the prevention of sexually transmitted infections (STIs)?

   _____

   _____

3. What is the role of the licensed practical nurse/licensed vocational nurse (LPN/LVN) with a woman having a pelvic examination?

   _____

   _____

   _____

   _____

VOCABULARY

Complete the following sentences with the correct term from the chapter.

1. A _____ may be done to view the inside of the uterus with an endoscope.
2. During some diagnostic procedures, a body cavity is filled with carbon dioxide to make it easier for the physician to view structures. This is called _____.
3. A male patient should have a yearly _____ examination to detect prostate cancer.
4. Some men have excessive breast tissue, which is called _____.
5. If the urethral opening is on the underside of the penis, it is called _____.
6. Fluid in the scrotum is called a _____.
7. If the scrotum feels like a bag of worms when palpated, it is called a _____.
8. Another word for sexual desire is _____.
9. The beginning of menstruation in the female is called _____.
10. X-ray examination of the breasts is called _____.

ANATOMY AND PHYSIOLOGY

Label the structures of the male and female reproductive systems.

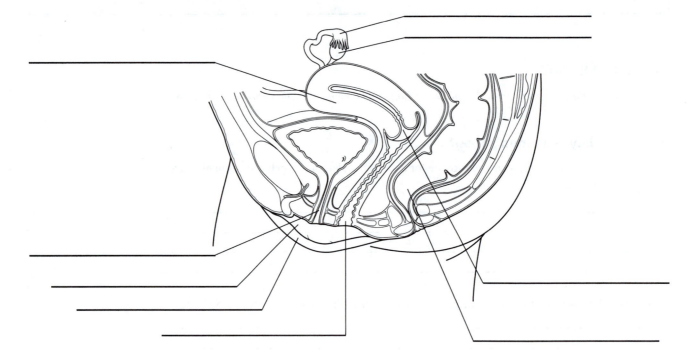

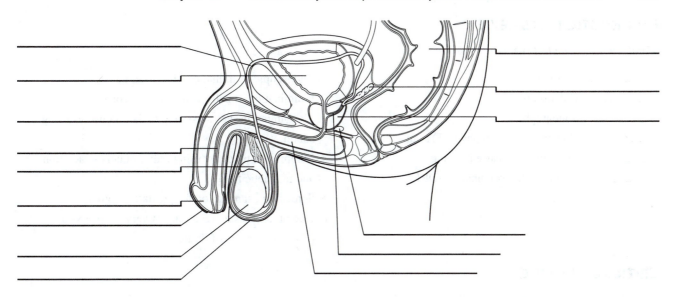

FEMALE REPRODUCTIVE STRUCTURES

Match the female reproductive structures with the correct descriptive statement.

1. _____ Fallopian tube

2. _____ Myometrium

3. _____ Bartholin glands

4. _____ Vestibule

5. _____ Endometrium

6. _____ Ovarian follicle

7. _____ Corpus luteum

1. Site of development of an ovum

2. Becomes the maternal side of the placenta

3. Contains the urethral and vaginal openings

4. Secretes progesterone and estrogen after ovulation

5. The usual site of fertilization

6. Secretes mucus at the vaginal orifice

7. Contracts for labor and delivery

MALE REPRODUCTIVE SYSTEM

Number the following in proper sequence with respect to the pathway sperm travel from their site of origin.

_____ Ejaculatory duct

_____ Epididymis

_____ Urethra

_____ Testes

_____ Ductus deferens

DIAGNOSTIC TESTS REVIEW

Match the following tests with their descriptions.

1. _____ Cytology
2. _____ Colposcopy
3. _____ Sonography
4. _____ Computed tomography (CT) scan
5. _____ Magnetic resonance imaging
6. _____ Digital rectal examination (DRE)

1. Endoscopic examination of the vagina
2. Examination of cells using a microscope
3. Mapping of tissues according to their densities using sound waves
4. Mapping of tissue by using radiofrequency radiation and magnetic fields
5. Screening examination for prostate disorders
6. Computer-assisted recording of very precise x-ray pictures of layers of tissue

CRITICAL THINKING

Read the scenarios and answer the following questions.

1. Mr. White comes to see his health care provider for a yearly checkup. As you are taking his blood pressure, he says, "I don't need that rectal examination, do I? I had prostate surgery last year." How do you respond?

_____

_____

_____

_____

2. Mrs. Bitner has just returned from having an endoscopic examination. She says, "Something went wrong. I just know it. Look at my belly. I look like I'm 9 months pregnant." How do you respond?

_____

_____

_____

_____

_____

3. Ms. Wilson comes to the clinic and reports excessive vaginal discharge. While asking her some initial questions, you learn that she has multiple sex partners. What do you anticipate for her examination? What teaching is important?

_____

_____

_____

_____

4. Mr. Brown is being admitted to the hospital for complications of diabetes. While collecting initial data, you learn that, although he is married, he is no longer sexually active. How do you respond?

_____

_____

_____

_____

_____

_____

REVIEW QUESTIONS—CONTENT REVIEW

Choose the best answer unless directed otherwise.

1. Which of the following male reproductive structures carries semen through the penis to the exterior?
   1. Urethra
   2. Epididymis
   3. Ductus deferens
   4. Ejaculatory duct

2. Which layer of the uterus will become the maternal portion of the placenta?
   1. Myometrium
   2. Endometrium
   3. Epimetrium
   4. Serosa

3. Which of the following descriptions best describes the position of the uterus?
   1. Superior to the bladder with the fundus most anterior
   2. Anterior to the bladder with the cervix most inferior
   3. Inferior to the bladder with the cervix most superior
   4. Posterior to the bladder with the fundus most inferior

4. Which of the following hormones stimulates the mammary glands to produce milk after pregnancy?
   1. Progesterone
   2. Estrogen
   3. Oxytocin
   4. Prolactin

5. Strong contractions of the smooth muscle of the uterus for labor and delivery are brought about by which of the following hormones?
   1. Progesterone
   2. Follicle-stimulating hormone
   3. Oxytocin
   4. Luteinizing hormone

6. According to the American Cancer Society, how often should a 40-year-old woman have a mammogram done?
   1. Weekly
   2. Monthly
   3. Yearly
   4. Every 2 years

7. When should men over age 50 have digital rectal examinations?
   1. Weekly
   2. Monthly
   3. Every other month
   4. During yearly physician visit

REVIEW QUESTIONS—TEST PREPARATION

Choose the best answer unless directed otherwise.

8. A patient being prepared for cystourethrography asks what is going to be done to him. Which is the best explanation by the nurse?
   1. "The doctor will put a tiny endoscope into your bladder."
   2. "You will have a catheter put in, then a dye will be injected and x-rays will be taken."
   3. "You will have a small needle inserted through your lower abdomen and into your bladder."
   4. "You will have an intravenous injection of dye; then x-rays will be taken as it travels through your kidneys."

9. The nurse is helping a woman prepare for a routine Papanicolaou (Pap) smear. Which of the following actions should the nurse take?
   1. Give the woman an enema.
   2. Ask the woman to empty her bladder.
   3. Ask the woman to take a deep breath and hold it.
   4. Set out a suture tray and local anesthetic.

10. A nurse is teaching breast self-examination. Which of the following positions would the nurse advise the patient to use for a portion of the exam?
    1. Supine
    2. Sims
    3. Kneeling
    4. Fowler

11. A woman receives notice that her screening mammogram is abnormal, and she is instructed to schedule diagnostic scans. The woman calls the office and asks the nurse, "Can you please tell me why I need more tests?" The nurse will base the response on which of the following understandings?
    1. A mammogram is able to diagnose cancerous lesions.
    2. Mammograms are unable to show lesions in breast tissue.
    3. A mammogram can show only breast cysts, not cancers.
    4. Many things can cause shadows on a mammogram besides cancer.

12. A nurse practitioner completes a wet-mount specimen on a patient with a suspected sexually transmitted infection and then leaves the room. As the assisting licensed practical nurse prepares to take the slide to the lab, the patient says, "I'm really scared that I have something serious. What do you think I should do?" Which response is best?
    1. Sit next to the patient and say, "What frightens you the most?"
    2. Stand at the foot of the examination table and say, "There is nothing to be worried about until we get the test results."
    3. Give the patient time to verbalize concerns, then advise that she have her partner tested.
    4. Touch her lightly on the arm and say, "Let me get this slide to the lab; then I'll come back and we'll talk."

CHAPTER 42
Nursing Care of Women With Reproductive System Disorders

Name: _____	
Date: _____	
Course: _____	
Instructor: _____	

AUDIO CASE STUDY
Mrs. Franklin and Total Abdominal Hysterectomy

Listen to the audio case study available on Davis Edge and then answer the following questions.

1. What problems did Mrs. Franklin have that could be treated by Michelle, her student nurse, following her hysterectomy?

   _____

   _____

2. What interventions did Michelle provide for Mrs. Franklin's constipation? What other interventions can be tried if the initial treatments do not work?

   _____

   _____

   _____

   _____

3. Should Michelle be concerned about the drainage on Mrs. Franklin's dressing? What should she watch for that would need to be reported to the health care provider (HCP)?

   _____

   _____

   _____

   _____

VOCABULARY

Match the term with its definition.

1. _____ Imperforate
2. _____ Colporrhaphy
3. _____ Dysmenorrhea
4. _____ Cryotherapy
5. _____ Agenesis
6. _____ Dyspareunia
7. _____ Cystocele
8. _____ Rectocele
9. _____ Anteversion
10. _____ Oophorectomy

1. Bladder sags into vaginal space
2. Painful menstruation
3. Not having expected opening
4. Surgical repair of a part of the vagina
5. Undeveloped
6. Rectum sags into the vagina
7. Painful intercourse
8. Forward turning
9. Removal of the ovaries
10. Freezing of tissue

BREAST SURGERIES

Match the following breast surgery terms with their descriptions.

1. _____ Mastopexy
2. _____ Mastectomy
3. _____ Reduction mammoplasty
4. _____ Augmentation mammoplasty
5. _____ Reconstructive mammoplasty

1. Surgery to remove a breast
2. Surgery to increase the size of the breasts
3. Surgery to decrease the size of the breasts
4. Surgery to rebuild a breast after mastectomy
5. Surgery to change the position of the breasts

MENSTRUAL DISORDERS

Match the following menstrual disorders with their definitions.

1. _____ Amenorrhea
2. _____ Menorrhagia
3. _____ Dysmenorrhea
4. _____ Polymenorrhea
5. _____ Hypomenorrhea

1. Difficult or painful menstruation
2. Menses more often than every 21 days
3. Passing more than 80 mL of blood per menses
4. Less than expected amount of menstrual bleeding
5. Absence of menstrual periods for 6 months or three previous cycle lengths once cycles have been established

MASTECTOMY CARE

Identify six errors in the following scenario and write the correct nursing care steps in the space provided.

You are assigned to care for Mrs. Joseph, who is 1-day postoperative following a right radical mastectomy. You know that she is not anxious because she had a left mastectomy a year ago and knows everything to expect. You listen to her breath sounds and find them clear, so it is not necessary to have her cough and deep breathe. You encourage her to lie on her right side to prevent bleeding. You use her right arm for blood pressures because both arms are affected and the right one is more convenient. You also encourage her to avoid use of her right arm to prevent injury to the surgical site. You provide a balanced diet and plenty of fluids to aid in her recovery.

1. _____
   _____
   _____
   _____

2. _____
   _____
   _____

3. _____
   _____
   _____

4. _____
   _____
   _____

5. _____
   _____
   _____

6. _____
   _____
   _____

CRITICAL THINKING

Read the following case study and answer the questions.

A 21-year-old female college student comes in to the physician's office where you work and comments with evident frustration that she has a yeast infection again. She has type 1 diabetes mellitus and takes her insulin routinely. However, she seldom tests her blood glucose level, because, she says, "I don't have time to mess with that stuff as often as I should." She comments that every time she goes home on weekends to visit her parents (a 3-hour bus trip), she develops a very uncomfortable vaginal yeast infection.

1. What factors may be contributing to her frequent yeast overgrowths? _____
   _____
   _____
   _____
   _____
   _____
   _____

2. What suggestions can you give her to help prevent this problem? _____
   _____
   _____
   _____
   _____
   _____
   _____
   _____
   _____
   _____
   _____

REVIEW QUESTIONS—CONTENT REVIEW

Choose the best answer unless directed otherwise.

1. How will a douche affect a vaginal examination to determine the type of pathogen present?
   1. A douche will help clear the area for better visualization.
   2. A douche does not affect the outcome negatively or positively.
   3. Douching can wash away evidence of the pathogen, making diagnosis difficult.
   4. Douching is recommended before the examination to neutralize the pH.

2. Which of the following is a known risk factor for cervical cancer?
   1. Tight clothing
   2. A high-sodium diet
   3. Multiple sexual partners
   4. Beginning sexual activity late in life

3. Which of the following is a risk factor for development of breast cancer?
   1. Late menarche
   2. High-fat diet
   3. Early menopause
   4. Early first pregnancy

REVIEW QUESTIONS—TEST PREPARATION

Choose the best answer unless directed otherwise.

4. Which of the following lifestyle habits are most likely to increase premenstrual syndrome symptoms? **Select all that apply.**
   1. Drinking alcohol
   2. Smoking
   3. Drinking coffee
   4. Eating a low-sodium diet
   5. Avoiding exercise before menses

5. A nurse is teaching a patient about use of a condom with spermicide for contraception. Which statement by the patient indicates the need for further teaching?
   1. "This method will be affordable."
   2. "I am glad that barrier methods are 100% effective."
   3. "I'm glad there are fewer side effects than there are with the pill."
   4. "I know that my husband and I will need to be diligent to use the method all the time."

6. Place in correct priority order the following nursing diagnoses for the woman who has just had a mastectomy for breast cancer.
   1. *Risk for Ineffective Peripheral Tissue Perfusion*
   2. *Ineffective Coping*
   3. *Ineffective Breathing Pattern*
   4. *Anxiety*

7. Which of the following nursing interventions will help prevent swelling after a radical mastectomy with lymph node removal?
   1. Restricting all movement of the affected arm
   2. Raising the affected arm above the heart on pillows
   3. Applying warm, moist heat to the arm
   4. Holding the arm close to the body with a sling

8. A patient who had a total hysterectomy 4 days ago for endometrial cancer learns that she has metastases to her lungs. When asked about her plans after discharge, she answers sharply that she "cannot plan for any future, because there isn't going to be any!" She then starts to cry. Which of the following nursing diagnoses best fits this situation?
   1. *Grieving*
   2. *Disturbed Body Image*
   3. *Disturbed Sleep Pattern*
   4. *Ineffective Health Maintenance*

9. A patient with breast cancer is being treated with tamoxifen citrate, which deprives cancer cells of the estrogen that makes them grow. This is an example of which mode of therapy?
   1. Hormonal antagonist therapy
   2. Radiation therapy
   3. Cytotoxic chemotherapy
   4. Biological response modifier therapy

10. A 38-year-old patient had a reduction mammoplasty 4 days ago. When changing her dressing, the home health care nurse notes redness, swelling, and some thick yellow drainage escaping from areas of the incision line around her left nipple. Which of the following nursing interventions is appropriate?
    1. Monitor it for 24 hours, and, if there is no improvement, notify the registered nurse or physician.
    2. Inform the patient that the incision is not healing properly and that she should see her physician as soon as possible.
    3. Clean the incision with normal saline, redress it, and recheck it the following day.
    4. Promptly report the situation to the supervisor or physician, and document it in the patient's chart.

CHAPTER 43
Nursing Care of Male Patients With Genitourinary Disorders

Name:	
Date:	
Course:	
Instructor:	

AUDIO CASE STUDY

Listen to the audio case study available on Davis Edge and then answer the following questions.

Mr. Poole and Transurethral Resection of the Prostate

1. What is the purpose of doing "serial urines" following prostate procedures?

_____

_____

_____

_____

2. What factors can increase risk of bleeding following a transurethral resection of the prostate (TURP)?

_____

_____

_____

_____

3. What is the purpose of a belladonna and opium suppository?

_____

_____

_____

_____

VOCABULARY

Fill in the blanks in the following sentences with terms from the chapter.

1. When semen goes into the bladder during intercourse, it is called _____ ejaculation.
2. An erection that lasts too long is called _____.
3. _____ is the term used to describe uncircumcised foreskin that cannot be extended over the head of the penis.
4. _____ is a cottage cheese–like secretion made by the gland of the foreskin.
5. Surgical removal of the foreskin is called _____.
6. _____ is a birth condition in which one or both of the testicles have not descended into the scrotum.
7. Inflammation or infection of a testicle is called _____.
8. The correct term for male impotence is _____.
9. A _____ is varicose veins of the scrotum.
10. Surgical interruption of the vas deferens as a method of birth control is called a _____.

DISORDERS OF THE MALE REPRODUCTIVE SYSTEM

Match the disorder with its definition.

1. _____ Benign prostatic hypertrophy (BPH)
2. _____ Hydronephrosis
3. _____ Hematuria
4. _____ Peyronie disease
5. _____ Priapism
6. _____ Epididymitis
7. _____ Infertility
8. _____ Orchitis
9. _____ Dysuria
10. _____ Reflux

1. Blood in the urine
2. Curved penis
3. Noncancerous overgrowth of prostate tissue
4. Inability to reproduce
5. Distention of kidney with retained urine
6. Inflammation of the testicles
7. Inflammation or infection of the tube where sperm matures
8. Painful or difficult urination
9. Backward flow of urine
10. Prolonged erection

ERECTILE DYSFUNCTION REVIEW

Unscramble the following causes of erectile dysfunction.

1. aeiioctdmn _____
2. sssrte _____
3. eeiophysnntr _____
4. PRUT _____
5. threa flraeiu _____
6. tiellpum lersssoic _____

CRITICAL THINKING

Read the following case study and answer the questions.

Mr. Washington is a 62-year-old retired teacher who comes to the urgent care center reporting that he "can't pass water."

1. What initial questions do you ask to further assess Mr. Washington's problem?

   _____

   _____

   _____

   _____

   _____

   _____

2. What do you think is happening?

   _____

   _____

   _____

   _____

   _____

3. What care do you anticipate as the physician examines him?

   _____

   _____

   _____

   _____

   _____

   _____

4. What can result if the problem continues untreated?

   _____

   _____

   _____

   Mr. Washington is transferred to the local hospital, where BPH is confirmed. He is scheduled for a TURP. He asks the nurse, "What's a TURP?"

5. How can the nurse explain a TURP to Mr. Washington?

   _____

   _____

   _____

   _____

6. After surgery, Mr. Washington has a three-way Foley catheter. What is the purpose of this type of catheter? How should the nurse total intake and output at the end of the shift?

   _____

   _____

   _____

   _____

   _____

7. Bladder spasms are common after TURP. How will the nurse know if this is happening? What interventions will help?

   _____

   _____

   _____

   _____

   _____

8. Mr. Washington is discharged. The next day he calls the nursing unit and says in a panicky voice, "I just wet my pants! I can't hold my urine! This is worse than not being able to go at all!" How should the nurse respond? What can Mr. Washington do?

   _____

   _____

   _____

   _____

   _____

   _____

REVIEW QUESTIONS—CONTENT REVIEW

Choose the best answer unless directed otherwise.

1. Which of the following nursing actions is most appropriate when doing perineal care on an uncircumcised male patient?
   1. Leave the foreskin retracted so air can keep the area dry.
   2. Do not retract the foreskin during washing.
   3. Replace the foreskin over the head of the penis after washing.
   4. Use alcohol and a cotton swab to clean under the foreskin.

2. What should be included when teaching young men to detect testicular cancer early?
   1. Monthly testicular self-examination
   2. Yearly digital rectal examination
   3. Annual physician examination
   4. Annual ultrasonography

REVIEW QUESTIONS—TEST PREPARATION

Choose the best answer unless directed otherwise.

3. The nurse completes a nursing history on a patient admitted for a transurethral resection of the prostate. Which symptoms of benign prostatic hyperplasia does the nurse expect the patient to report? **Select all that apply.**
   1. A feeling of incomplete bladder emptying after voiding
   2. Difficulty maintaining an erection
   3. Difficulty urinating
   4. Grossly bloody urine
   5. Pain in the lower back that radiates to the hips during urination
   6. Nocturia

4. A patient tells his nurse that he has delayed having a transurethral resection of the prostate because he is afraid it will affect his sexual function. Which response by the nurse is most appropriate?
   1. "Don't worry about sterility. Sperm production is not affected by this surgery."
   2. "Would you like some information about implants used for impotence?"
   3. "This type of surgery rarely affects the ability to have an erection or ejaculation."
   4. "There are many methods of sexual expression that are alternatives to sexual intercourse."

5. A patient returns from surgery following a transurethral resection of the prostate with a three-way Foley catheter and continuous bladder irrigation. Postoperative orders include morphine 5 to 10 mg intramuscularly every 3 hours as needed for pain, belladonna and opium suppository every 4 hours as needed, and strict input and output. The patient reports painful bladder spasms, and the nurse observes blood-tinged urine on the sheets. Which action should the nurse take first?
   1. Administer the morphine.
   2. Administer the belladonna and opium suppository.
   3. Warm the irrigation solution to body temperature.
   4. Notify the physician STAT.

6. A patient who has just had a transurethral resection of the prostate asks his nurse to explain why he has to have the bladder irrigation because it seems to increase his pain. Which of the following explanations by the nurse is best?
   1. "The bladder irrigation is needed to stop the bleeding in the bladder."
   2. "Antibiotics are being administered into the bladder to prevent infection."
   3. "The irrigation is needed to keep the catheter from becoming occluded by blood clots."
   4. "Normal production of urine is maintained with the irrigations until healing can occur."

7. A post–transurethral resection of the prostate patient experiences dribbling following removal of his catheter. Which action should the nurse take?
   1. Encourage him to restrict fluid intake to 1,000 mL/day.
   2. Teach him to perform Kegel exercises 10 to 20 times per hour.
   3. Reinsert the Foley catheter until he regains urinary control.
   4. Reassure him that incontinence never lasts more than a few days.

8. A 36-year-old man is scheduled for a unilateral orchiectomy for treatment of testicular cancer. He is withdrawn and does not interact with the nurse. Which action is most appropriate?
   1. Identify the problem with a nursing diagnosis of *Impaired Communication* related to the diagnosis of cancer.
   2. Set a patient outcome that the patient will verbalize his concerns about his diagnosis.
   3. Ask the patient whether he is worried about future sexual functioning.
   4. Say, "You seem quiet. Are you feeling concerned about your diagnosis or treatment?"

9. A 28-year-old man is diagnosed with acute epididymitis. For which of the following symptoms should the nurse assess?
   1. Burning and pain on urination
   2. Severe tenderness and swelling in the scrotum
   3. Foul-smelling ejaculate and severe scrotal swelling
   4. Foul-smelling urine and pain on urination

10. A man with a history of diabetes and chronic lung disease is admitted to the hospital with prostate cancer. He has all the following symptoms. Which should the nurse address first?
    1. Fever of 101°F (38.3°C)
    2. Respiratory rate of 36 per minute
    3. Difficulty urinating
    4. Painful legs and feet

11. The nurse is providing care for a patient scheduled for a vasectomy. Which of the following statements indicates further teaching is necessary?
    1. "I will need to have my testosterone levels checked periodically to ensure the success of the surgery."
    2. "Another method of birth control should be used for the next 3 months."
    3. "The amount and color of my ejaculate should be the same as before surgery."
    4. "I'll have to bring a sample of semen back for evaluation after the surgery."

CHAPTER 44
Nursing Care of Patients With Sexually Transmitted Infections

Name: _____	
Date: _____	
Course: _____	
Instructor: _____	

AUDIO CASE STUDY

Listen to the audio case study available on Davis Edge and then answer the following questions.

Janis Works at the STI Clinic

1. Janis would not allow Hannah's boyfriend to come into the examination room. Why was this important?

   _____

   _____

   _____

   _____

2. What can be the consequence of having sex with someone new without that person first being tested for sexually transmitted infections (STIs)?

   _____

   _____

   _____

   _____

3. What are symptoms of a herpes simplex virus type 2 (HSV-2) infection?

   _____

   _____

   _____

   _____

VOCABULARY

Match the term with its definition.

1. _____ Condylomatous
2. _____ Gumma
3. _____ Chancre
4. _____ Cytotoxic
5. _____ Herpetic
6. _____ Puerperal

1. Relating to herpes
2. Rubbery tumor
3. Red ulcer from syphilis
4. Wart-like
5. Poison to cells
6. Time following childbirth

INFLAMMATORY DISORDERS

Match the following inflammation words with their definitions.

1. _____ Proctitis
2. _____ Urethritis
3. _____ Cervicitis
4. _____ Endometritis
5. _____ Conjunctivitis

1. Inflammation of the rectum and anus
2. Inflammation of the cervix
3. Inflammation of the urethra
4. Inflammation of parts of the eye
5. Inflammation of the lining of the uterus

BARRIER METHODS FOR SAFER SEX

List the teaching that should accompany each of the following barriers against STIs.

1. Male condoms _____

_____

_____

_____

_____

_____

_____

2. Female condoms _____

_____

_____

_____

_____

_____

3. Cervical caps or diaphragms _____

_____

_____

4. Rubber gloves, rubber dental dams, or split (opened) male condoms _____

_____

_____

_____

_____

_____

5. Double condoms _____

_____

_____

_____

_____

_____

CRITICAL THINKING

Read the following case study and answer the questions.

James, 32 years old, arrives at an outpatient clinic requesting STI testing for him and his fiancée. You learn that he met his fiancée through an international dating agency and that she has come to the United States to marry him. She does not speak English. He asks you to give him the paperwork for both of them to get the blood test for STIs "just to make sure they don't have anything contagious." He seems in a hurry and asks if they can have their blood drawn first and then he could come back in an hour or two and see the doctor for the results for both of them.

1. What misunderstandings does James have about STI diagnosis?

_____

_____

_____

_____

_____

_____

2. Legally and ethically, does James have a right to be told his fiancée's test results?

_____

_____

_____

_____

_____

_____

3. What procedures should occur before any testing is done?

_____

_____

_____

_____

_____

4. Is James likely to get his answer about whether either he or his fiancée has a contagious STI today?

_____

_____

_____

_____

_____

REVIEW QUESTIONS—CONTENT REVIEW

Choose the best answer unless directed otherwise.

1. Which of the following sexually transmitted infections is associated with gummas?
   1. Gonorrhea
   2. Herpes simplex virus
   3. Trichomoniasis
   4. Syphilis

2. Which virus causes genital warts?
   1. Cytomegalovirus
   2. Herpes simplex virus type 2
   2. Human papillomavirus
   3. Human immunodeficiency virus

REVIEW QUESTIONS—TEST PREPARATION

Choose the best answer unless directed otherwise.

3. A 36-year-old woman who has had no prenatal care comes into the hospital in active labor with her fourth child. She has vesicles evident on her perineum. Which of the following nursing actions are appropriate to protect the unborn baby and the staff? **Select all that apply.**
   1. Maintain standard precautions.
   2. Reprimand the mother for putting her baby at risk for herpes.
   3. Prepare for the possibility that the baby may be delivered by cesarean section.
   4. Notify the obstetrician or nurse midwife about the vesicles as soon as possible.
   5. Apply antibiotic ointment to the vesicles.
   6. Place the mother in reverse isolation.

4. A 23-year-old woman is seen at an outpatient clinic for a routine Papanicolaou (Pap) smear. When questioned, she states she is deciding whether to engage in sexual activity with a man she is just getting to know. She asks how she can tell if he has a sexually transmitted infection. Which response by the nurse is best?
   1. "If the man appears clean and has been conscientious about using condoms, he is likely infection free."
   2. "Look carefully for signs of lesions before engaging in sexual activity."
   3. "Be sure to use either a male or female condom to protect against possible transmission of infection."
   4. "An examination by a physician with diagnostic testing is the only way to know if he is infection free."

5. A college student goes to the college clinic and asks the best way to avoid contracting a sexually transmitted infection. The nurse provides the clinic's standard sexually transmitted infection teaching. Which statement by the student indicates the need for additional instruction?
   1. "There is no guarantee that I won't contract a sexually transmitted infection if I choose to be sexually active."
   2. "Abstinence is the only sure way to avoid a sexually transmitted infection."
   3. "If I use a condom with spermicide, I will be safer than if I don't use one."
   4. "If I question my partner about past sexual encounters, I can avoid sexually transmitted infections."

6. While bathing an 82-year-old man hospitalized with pneumonia, a nurse notes an ulcerated area on his penis. What action should the nurse take first?
   1. Report the ulcer to the admitting care provider.
   2. Teach the man about sexually transmitted infection prevention.
   3. Ask the man if he has a history of syphilis.
   4. Clean the ulcer; reporting is not necessary because a sexually transmitted infection is unlikely in a man this age.

7. A patient has cloudy penile discharge. For which additional symptoms of urethritis should the nurse assess?
   1. Throat or rectal infection
   2. Chancres or vesicles on the genitals
   3. Painful and frequent urination
   4. Oliguria and flank pain

8. A woman with pelvic inflammatory disease says she has lower abdominal pain. Which action should the nurse take first?
   1. Have her rate her pain on a 0 to 10 scale.
   2. Administer antibiotics as ordered.
   3. Administer an analgesic as ordered.
   4. Teach the patient about causes and prevention of sexually transmitted infections.

9. A nurse needs to administer an intramuscular injection of 2.4 million units of penicillin G. It is supplied in a vial of 5 million units of powder for injection. Instructions state to dilute with 8 mL of sterile water. How many mL should the nurse draw up?

   _____

10. The nurse receives a phone call from a client who reports engaging in recent sexual activity with a partner who just informed her that he has herpes. Which of the following statements by the nurse is best?
    1. "How long has your partner had herpes?"
    2. "Did you notice any rash or other lesions on his face or genitalia?"
    3. "You need to use a diaphragm if you engage in sexual intercourse with him again."
    4. "If you notice flu-like symptoms, symptoms of a bladder infection, or vaginal drainage within the next 2 weeks you need to be seen right away."

CHAPTER 45
Musculoskeletal Function and Assessment

Name: _____	
Date: _____	
Course: _____	
Instructor: _____	

AUDIO CASE STUDY

Listen to the audio case study available on Davis Edge and then answer the following questions.

Tony and Fracture Care

1. What are primary and secondary surveys?

   _____

   _____

   _____

   _____

   _____

2. What complications could develop in Evan from hitting the steering wheel in the accident?

   _____

   _____

3. What is examined during a neurovascular check on an extremity?

   _____

   _____

   _____

   _____

   _____

STRUCTURE OF NEUROMUSCULAR JUNCTION AND SARCOMERES

Label the structures from the following word list.

Acetylcholine (ACh) receptors
Motor neuron
Myofilaments
Sarcolemma
Sarcomere

Sarcoplasmic reticulum
Synaptic cleft
T tubule
Vesicles of acetylcholine (ACh)

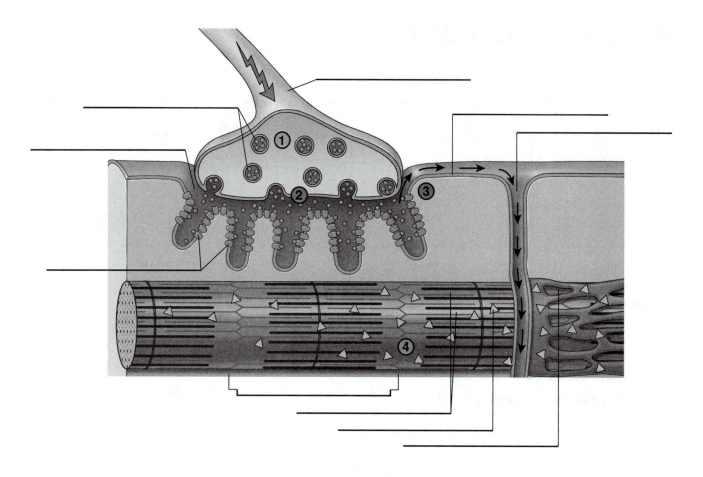

NEUROMUSCULAR JUNCTION

Match each part of the neuromuscular junction with the proper descriptions. Each part will have two correct answers.

1. _____ Synaptic cleft
2. _____ Axon terminal
3. _____ Sarcolemma

1. Contains the transmitter acetylcholine in vesicles
2. The cell membrane of the muscle fiber
3. The space between the muscle fiber and the motor neuron
4. Electrical impulse is sent over this.
5. Acetylcholine is released into this area.
6. Located at the end of the motor neuron

SYNOVIAL JOINTS

Match each part of a synovial joint with the correct function.

1. _____ Articular cartilage
2. _____ Joint capsule
3. _____ Synovial membrane
4. _____ Synovial fluid
5. _____ Bursae

1. Lines the joint capsule and secretes synovial fluid
2. Prevents friction within the joint cavity
3. Encloses the joint similar to a sleeve
4. Permit tendons to slide easily across a joint
5. Provides a smooth surface on the joint surfaces of bones

VOCABULARY

Match the word on the left with its definition on the right.

1. _____ Symphysis
2. _____ Ball and socket
3. _____ Hinge
4. _____ Articular
5. _____ Pivot
6. _____ Gliding
7. _____ Saddle
8. _____ Bursa
9. _____ Crepitation
10. _____ Synovitis

1. Movement in all planes
2. Rotation
3. Disk of fibrous cartilage between bones
4. Movement in one plane
5. Relating to a joint
6. Swollen synovial tissue within the joint
7. Small sacs of synovial fluid between joints and tendons
8. Movement in several planes
9. Side-to-side movement
10. Grating sound as joint or bone moves

DIAGNOSTIC TESTS

Match each diagnostic test to its appropriate description.

1. _____ X-ray
2. _____ Arthrogram
3. _____ Magnetic resonance imaging
4. _____ Arthroscopy
5. _____ Arthrocentesis
6. _____ Bone scan
7. _____ Serum alkaline phosphatase
8. _____ Serum calcium
9. _____ Serum phosphorus
10. _____ Dual energy x-ray absorptiometry
11. _____ Uric acid

1. Dye used to view joint structures (tendons, ligaments, cartilage)
2. Radio waves and magnetic field view of soft tissue
3. Bones appear as white areas
4. Insertion of a needle into a joint space to aspirate fluid, obtain a specimen, or instill medication
5. Endoscopy of joints with local or general anesthesia
6. Enzyme made by osteoblasts to mineralize bone
7. After injection, a radioisotope is taken up by bone and 2 hours later a camera scans the body front and back
8. End product of purine metabolism
9. Special x-ray evaluating bone density
10. Mineralizes bones and teeth
11. Stored in bone to make bone rigid

CRITICAL THINKING

Read the following case study and answer the questions.

Mr. John Allen, age 45, is in an automobile accident and comes to the emergency department with a fractured femur.

1. What data should the nurse collect in Mr. Allen's history?

   _____

   _____

   _____

2. What areas should Mr. Allen's physical examination focus on first?

   _____

   _____

   _____

3. What tests can the nurse anticipate will be performed for Mr. Allen?

   _____

   _____

   _____

4. What types of patient teaching should the nurse provide?

   _____

   _____

   _____

   _____

REVIEW QUESTIONS—CONTENT REVIEW

Choose the best answer unless directed otherwise.

1. Absorbing shock between adjacent vertebrae is the function of disks made of which of the following?
   1. Smooth muscle
   2. Synovial fluid
   3. Fibrous cartilage
   4. Adipose tissue

2. Which of the following is the transmitter at neuromuscular junctions?
   1. Sodium ions
   2. Acetylcholine
   3. A nerve impulse
   4. Cholinesterase

3. Muscles are attached to bones by which of the following?
   1. Tendons
   2. Ligaments
   3. Fascia
   4. Other muscles

4. Which of the following is the part of the brain that initiates muscle contraction?
   1. Parietal lobe
   2. Cerebellum
   3. Frontal lobe
   4. Temporal lobe

5. Which of the following organ systems are directly necessary for muscle contraction? **Select all that apply.**
   1. Circulatory system
   2. Digestive system
   3. Respiratory system
   4. Nervous system
   5. Sensory system

6. Which of the following is the function of synovial fluid in joints?
   1. Exchange nutrients
   2. Prevent friction
   3. Absorb water
   4. Wear away rough surfaces

REVIEW QUESTIONS—TEST PREPARATION

Choose the best answer unless directed otherwise.

7. The nurse is inspecting the knee of a patient who reports pain and stiffness. As the patient moves the knee, the nurse hears a grating sound. The nurse correctly documents the grating sound as which of the following?
   1. Friction rub
   2. Crepitation
   3. Effusion
   4. Subcutaneous emphysema

8. What actions should the nurse take after observing a joint that has a grating sound with movement? **Select all that apply.**
   1. Abduct the extremity.
   2. Adduct the extremity.
   3. Immediately stop joint movement.
   4. Flex the joint.
   5. Protect the joint.
   6. Maintain joint immobilization.

9. The nurse is gathering functional data on a patient with arthritis. The nurse would collect data in which of these areas? **Select all that apply.**
   1. Ability to feed self
   2. Appearance of joints
   3. Bathing practices
   4. Dressing ability
   5. Pain level
   6. Response to treatment

10. Following a patient's bone biopsy, the nurse inspects the biopsy site. The nurse is monitoring for what complication that may occur immediately following a biopsy?
    1. Joint dislocation
    2. Crepitation
    3. Infection
    4. Hematoma formation

11. The nurse would evaluate the patient as requiring further teaching if the patient stated which of these serum blood tests is elevated in gout? **Select all that apply.**
    1. Alkaline phosphatase
    2. Calcium
    3. Creatine kinase
    4. Myoglobin
    5. Phosphorus
    6. Uric acid

12. A patient is scheduled to have magnetic resonance imaging of the abdomen. Patient data collected includes no known drug allergies, history of hypertension, surgical history of appendectomy, and left cardiac permanent pacemaker implantation. Mark the area in which the contraindication to the magnetic resonance imaging is located that the nurse will report to the health care provider.

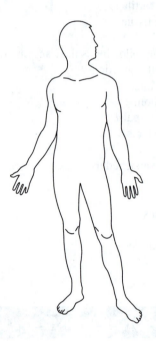

CHAPTER 46
Nursing Care of Patients With Musculoskeletal and Connective Tissue Disorders

Name:	
Date:	
Course:	
Instructor:	

AUDIO CASE STUDY

Listen to the audio case study available on Davis Edge and then answer the following questions.

Alex and Osteomyelitis

1. What is a complication of an open fracture?

   _____

   _____

   _____

2. How can the nurse help to prevent a debilitating bone infection?

   _____

   _____

   _____

3. What treatment was used for Alex's phantom pain?

   _____

   _____

   _____

VOCABULARY

Fill in the blank with the word that is formed by the word building.

1. _____ arthro (joint) + itis (inflammation)
2. _____ arthro (joint) + plasty (creation of)
3. _____ synovia (synovial fluid or tissue) + itis (inflammation)
4. _____ arthro (joint) + centesis (puncture of a cavity)
5. _____ hyper (excessive) + uric (uric acid) + emia (in blood)
6. _____ vascul (blood vessel) + itis (inflammation)
7. _____ a (without) + vascular (blood) + necrosis (death)
8. _____ re (again) + plant (to plant) + tion (process)
9. _____ hemi (half) + pelv (pelvis) + ectomy (removal of)
10. _____ fascia (fibrous tissue) + otomy (opening into)
11. _____ osteo (bone) + sarco (flesh) + oma (tumor)
12. _____ osteo (bone) + myel (bone marrow) + itis (inflammation)

FRACTURES

Match the type of fracture with its definition.

1. _____ More than two fragments that appear to float
2. _____ At right angle to bone
3. _____ Splintered and bent, occurring mainly in children
4. _____ More than two fragments driven into each other
5. _____ Extends into articular surface
6. _____ Runs along axis of bone
7. _____ Oblique fracture line
8. _____ Spontaneous fracture from bone disease
9. _____ Fracture twists around shaft of bone
10. _____ From repeated stress (e.g., jogging)

1. Transverse
2. Stress
3. Spiral
4. Pathological
5. Oblique
6. Longitudinal
7. Interarticular
8. Impacted
9. Greenstick
10. Comminuted

PROSTHESIS CARE EDUCATION

Indicate whether the statement is true or false, and correct false statements.

1. _____ Replace worn shoes with ones of a different height and type.
2. _____ Clean the prosthesis socket with alcohol and water, and dry it completely.
3. _____ Replace worn inserts and liners when they become too soiled to clean.
4. _____ Use garters to keep socks or stockings in place.
5. _____ Oil the mechanical parts as instructed by the physician.

HEALTH PROMOTION FOR PATIENTS WITH GOUT

Fill in the blanks.

1. Avoid high _____ foods, such as organ meats, shellfish, and oily fish, such as _____.
2. _____ alcohol.
3. Drink plenty of _____, especially water.
4. Avoid all forms of _____ and medications containing _____.
5. _____ diuretics.
6. Avoid excessive physical or emotional _____.
7. Consider drinking _____ juice.

CRITICAL THINKING

Complete the nursing care plan for the nursing diagnosis Impaired Physical Mobility *for a patient with a total hip replacement.*

NURSING DIAGNOSIS
Impaired Physical Mobility *related to hip precautions and surgical pain*

Interventions	Rationale	Evaluation
• _____ _____ _____	• Activity is restricted due to hip precautions and weight-bearing limitations.	• _____ _____ _____
• Monitor the patient for and take measures to prevent complications of immobility.	• _____ _____ _____	• Is the patient free from complications of immobility?
• Turn patient every 2 hours to the side ordered and check skin.		
• _____ _____ _____ _____		
• _____ _____ _____ _____		
• _____ _____ _____ _____		
• _____ _____ _____ _____		
• _____ _____ _____ _____		
• Mobilize the patient as soon as possible as prescribed.		

REVIEW QUESTIONS—CONTENT REVIEW

Choose the best answer unless directed otherwise.

1. Which of the following is the recommended protocol for caring for a severed body part that may be replanted? **Select all that apply.**
   1. Cover it with a warm, dry towel.
   2. Wrap it in a clean, moist cloth.
   3. Place it directly on dry ice.
   4. Wrap it in a dry, sterile dressing.
   5. Seal in plastic bag.
   6. Place it in ice.

2. Which of these laboratory values should the nurse monitor for a patient with gout?
   1. Blood urea nitrogen
   2. Creatinine
   3. Uric acid
   4. Cholesterol

REVIEW QUESTIONS—TEST PREPARATION

Choose the best answer unless directed otherwise.

3. A patient is in skin traction using a foam boot with Velcro fasteners for a fractured hip. The nurse would document this type of skin traction as which of the following?
   1. Gardner tongs
   2. Buck traction
   3. Crutchfield tongs
   4. Steinmann pin

4. A patient sustains a closed fracture of the right tibia and is placed in a long-leg plaster cast, which is still damp. Which of the following methods should the nurse use to move the cast to prevent complications?
   1. Have patient reposition own leg.
   2. Use palms to move the cast.
   3. Use fingertips to grasp cast.
   4. Do not move the cast until it is dry.

5. A patient is being treated with gold therapy for rheumatoid arthritis. Which of the following interventions is essential when gold therapy is started? **Select all that apply.**
   1. Remove all metal objects patient is wearing.
   2. Check allergies to iodine.
   3. Give a test dose of gold.
   4. Plan a biweekly dosing schedule.
   5. Monitor the patient after the injection.
   6. Teach the patient to obtain daily weight.

6. The nurse is caring for a patient who has a fractured ankle in a cast. The patient has morphine 5 to 10 mg intramuscularly ordered every 3 to 4 hours. The patient received morphine 5 mg 2 hours and 45 minutes ago. The patient is rating the pain at 10 and moans that the leg hurts. Vital signs are within normal limits. The patient has good capillary refill. Which of the following actions is most appropriate for the nurse to take next?
   1. Apply ice to the cast.
   2. Notify the health care provider immediately.
   3. Remove the pillow under the cast.
   4. Prepare morphine 10 mg for administration.

7. The nurse turns a 2-day postoperative patient with a right total hip replacement using three pillows between the legs. The nurse later returns and finds the patient lying supine with legs crossed. Which of the following should the nurse immediately observe to determine whether a complication has developed?
   1. The right knee for crepitation
   2. The left leg for internal rotation
   3. The left leg for loss of function
   4. The right leg for shortening

8. The nurse provides discharge teaching for the patient with gout. The nurse would evaluate the patient as understanding if the patient says which of the following can be eaten? **Select all that apply.**
   1. Cod
   2. Chicken
   3. Eggs
   4. Liver
   5. Sardines
   6. Cherries

9. Which of the following medications should a patient with gout be encouraged to avoid in order to prevent a gout attack?
   1. Aspirin
   2. Acetaminophen
   3. Motrin
   4. Codeine
   5. Excedrin
   6. Percodan

10. The nurse is reviewing an erythrocyte sedimentation rate for a patient. Which of the following does the nurse understand is the purpose of this test?
    1. To identify the number of red blood cells the patient has
    2. To determine sedimentation found in red blood cells
    3. To identify the presence of systemic inflammation
    4. To diagnose various types of arthritis

11. Which patient data does the nurse recognize as a risk factor for a patient with a history of a pathological fracture? **Select all that apply.**
    1. History of falling
    2. Paget disease
    3. Jogging
    4. Cancer
    5. Osteoporosis
    6. Daily carbonated beverage intake

12. Which of the following symptoms would the nurse most likely be told was the first symptom that caused a patient with rheumatoid arthritis to seek health care?
    1. Cold intolerance
    2. Stiff, sore joints
    3. Shortness of breath
    4. Crepitation

13. The nurse teaches the patient, who has risk factors for osteoporosis, prevention methods. The nurse evaluates the patient as understanding the teaching if the patient states lifestyle changes will include which of these? **Select all that apply.**
    1. Daily walking
    2. Increased milk intake
    3. Limited dark green leafy vegetables
    4. Weight training
    5. Maintaining normal weight
    6. Calcium supplement

14. The nurse is to administer alendronate (Fosamax) to a patient. Which of the following actions should the nurse implement to safely administer the medication? **Select all that apply.**
    1. Verify allergies.
    2. Administer at bedtime.
    3. Give on an empty stomach.
    4. Give with 6 to 8 ounces of water only.
    5. After administration, wait 1 hour before giving other medication.
    6. Instruct patient to remain upright for 30 minutes.

15. The nurse is teaching the patient about contracture prevention after an above-the-knee amputation. The nurse evaluates the patient as requiring further teaching if the patient states which of these interventions should be used? **Select all that apply.**
    1. Lie prone for 30 minutes.
    2. Sit in chair for 2 hours.
    3. Elevate stump on pillow daily.
    4. Ensure stump lies flat on bed.
    5. Elevate head of bed during the day.
    6. Elevate foot of bed daily.

16. The nurse is collecting data on a patient who is experiencing an acute attack of gout. Mark the area where the nurse would inspect the patient for the most commonly occurring symptom of gout.

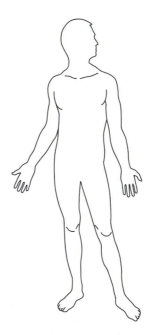

CHAPTER 47
Neurologic System Function, Assessment, and Therapeutic Measures

Name:	_____
Date:	_____
Course:	_____
Instructor:	_____

AUDIO CASE STUDY

Listen to the audio case study available on Davis Edge and then answer the following questions.

Mrs. Beason Passes Out

1. What are the basic parts of a neurological assessment that Betty performed?

   _____

   _____

2. Why did Betty ask if Mrs. Beason knew where she was?

   _____

   _____

3. What care and teaching would you provide for a patient having an angiogram?

   _____

   _____

   _____

   _____

   _____

   _____

   _____

   _____

4. Why was an angiogram planned for Mrs. Beason?

_____

_____

_____

VOCABULARY

Fill in the blank with the correct term.

1. Difficulty swallowing is called _____.

2. An _____ is a test that uses scalp electrodes to evaluate brain activity.

3. A patient might say his leg feels like it is asleep to describe _____.

4. Abnormal flexion posturing when eliciting best motor response is called _____ posturing.

5. Abnormal extension posturing when eliciting best motor response is called _____ posturing.

6. _____ is the term that describes unequal pupils.

7. Involuntary eye movement is called _____.

8. Permanent muscle contractions are called _____.

9. Difficulty speaking because of muscle dysfunction is called _____.

10. Patients who have difficulty speaking after a stroke are experiencing _____.

DIAGNOSTIC TESTS

Describe the procedure and nursing care before and after each of the following diagnostic tests used for neurological diagnoses. (See Davis Edge for complete descriptions.)

1. Myelogram _____

_____

_____

_____

_____

_____

_____

_____

_____

2. Electroencephalogram (EEG) _____

_____

_____

_____

_____

_____

_____

3. Lumbar puncture _____

_____

_____

_____

_____

_____

_____

_____

_____

4. Magnetic resonance imaging (MRI) _____

_____

_____

_____

_____

_____

_____

_____

5. Computed tomography (CT) scan _____

_____

_____

_____

_____

_____

_____

_____

_____

ANATOMY

Label the parts of the cerebrum.

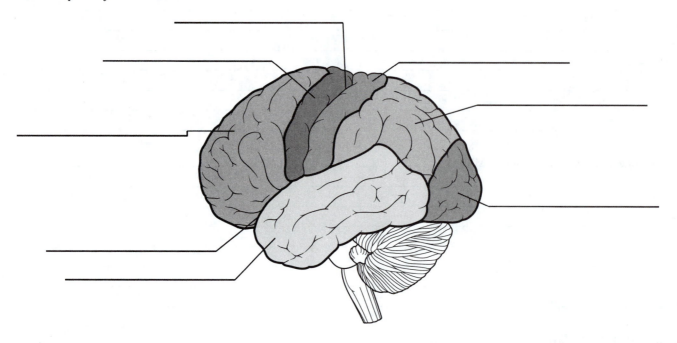

Label the parts of the neuron.

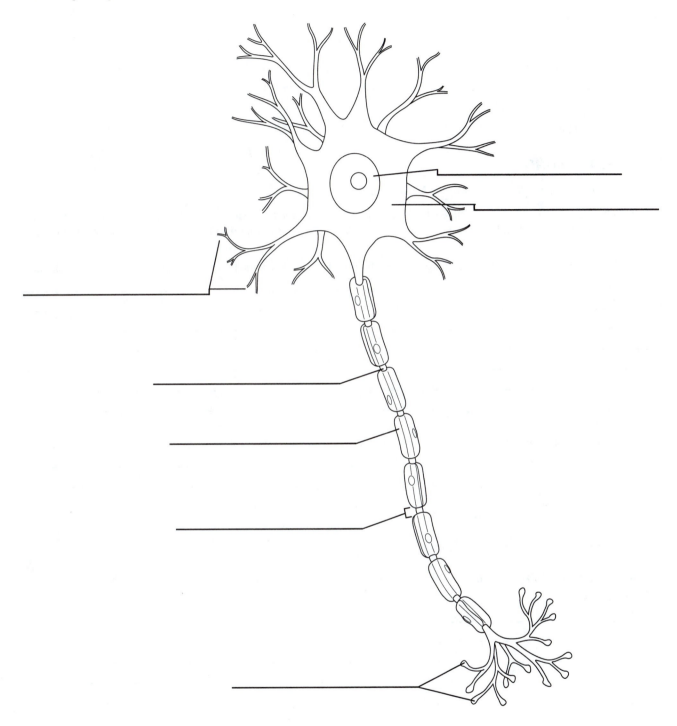

ANATOMY REVIEW

Match the part of the brain with the function it controls.

1. _____ Cerebrum

2. _____ Medulla oblongata

3. _____ Occipital lobe

4. _____ Cerebellum

5. _____ Temporal lobe

1. Vision center

2. Speech

3. Equilibrium and coordination

4. Respiratory center

5. Information storage

ASSESSMENT OF CRANIAL NERVES

Match the following assessment tools with the nerve to be tested.

1. _____ Cotton ball

2. _____ Snellen chart

3. _____ Use of hands to check neck/shoulder strength

4. _____ Tuning fork or whisper

5. _____ Tongue blade and cotton swab

1. Vestibulocochlear (VIII)

2. Accessory (XI)

3. Trigeminal (V)

4. Optic (II)

5. Vagus (X)

CRITICAL THINKING

Read the following case study and answer the following questions.

Mrs. Pickett is admitted to the nursing home where you work as a nurse. She had a stroke 2 weeks ago and is not strong enough to go to a rehabilitation facility. She has left-sided weakness. You collect admitting data to help determine her plan of care.

1. Mrs. Pickett tells you she needs to get up to go to the bathroom. What are some things you can do to determine if she is able to do this? _____

_____

_____

_____

_____

_____

2. Mrs. Pickett's first meal is served. What can you do to determine her ability to eat safely?_____

_____

_____

_____

_____

_____

3. Mrs. Pickett says, "Will you go to the kitchen and get me one of those cookies I like?" How do you determine whether she is confused? _____

_____

_____

_____

_____

4. Mrs. Pickett is weak on her left side. Why do you think her blood pressure will be more accurate in her right arm?

_____

_____

_____

REVIEW QUESTIONS—CONTENT REVIEW

Choose the best answer unless directed otherwise.

1. Which of the following parts of a neuron transmits impulses away from the cell body?
   1. Dendrite
   2. Axon
   3. Neurolemma
   4. Synapse

2. Which type of neuron transmits impulses from the central nervous system to the muscles and glands?
   1. Afferent
   2. Efferent

3. Which part of the brain controls breathing?
   1. Medulla oblongata
   2. Cerebellum
   3. Cerebrum
   4. Thalamus

4. When a neurologist asks a patient to smile, which cranial nerve is being tested?
   1. II, optic
   2. VII, facial
   3. X, vagus
   4. XI, accessory

5. The neurologist tests the fourth (trochlear) and sixth (abducens) cranial nerves together by having a patient do which of the following?
   1. Turn the head to the right and left.
   2. Identify whispering in the ears.
   3. Say "Aaaah."
   4. Follow a finger with the eyes.

6. Which of the following responses indicates sympathetic nervous system activation?
   1. Tachycardia, dilated pupils
   2. Increased peristalsis, abdominal cramping
   3. Hypoglycemia, headache
   4. Pupil constriction, bronchoconstriction

7. Which neurotransmitter mediates the sympathetic response?
   1. Acetylcholine
   2. Prostaglandin
   3. Norepinephrine
   4. Serotonin

REVIEW QUESTIONS—TEST PREPARATION

Choose the best answer unless directed otherwise.

8. Which of the following actions are controlled by nerves exiting from the cervical portion of the spinal cord? **Select all that apply.**
   1. Blinking
   2. Writing
   3. Sticking out the tongue
   4. Nodding
   5. Urinating

9. The nurse is assisting a patient to prepare for a lumbar puncture. Which of the following actions should the nurse take first?
   1. Administer enemas until clear.
   2. Remove all metal jewelry.
   3. Position the patient on the side.
   4. Remove the patient's dentures.

10. The nurse is caring for a patient with left-sided paresis and inability to walk following a stroke. Which intervention will help increase the possibility of the patient walking again?
    1. Have the family bring high-top tennis shoes for the patient to wear in bed.
    2. Administer muscle relaxants as ordered to maintain comfort.
    3. Position the patient to reduce pressure on bony prominences.
    4. Provide assistive devices so the patient can manage personal care independently.

11. The nurse knows that the patient understands instructions for getting magnetic resonance imaging when the patient makes which statement?
    1. "I will have a small Band-Aid on the puncture site."
    2. "I will need to wash my hair following it."
    3. "I should avoid eating or drinking for 4 hours after the procedure."
    4. "I should be sure to remove all metal jewelry."

12. The nurse is providing care for a patient scheduled for a computed tomography scan of the brain with contrast media. Which of the following statements should be included in the patient teaching? **Select all that apply.**
    1. "You will need to lie still for 1 to 2 hours during the exam."
    2. "Notify the staff if you have any nausea, sweating, or itching during the exam."
    3. "Mild sedation can be given if you become uncomfortable."
    4. "You may have a feeling of warmth throughout your body after the dye is injected."
    5. "The table may be moved to various positions during the test."
    6. "This test can't be used if you have any metal in your body."

13. The nurse is assessing the patient's cranial nerves. Mark the area where the nurse would focus assessment of the motor impulses from the glossopharyngeal and vagal nerves.

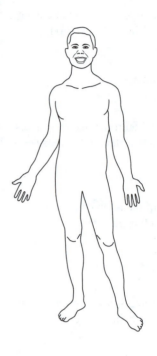

CHAPTER 48
Nursing Care of Patients With Central Nervous System Disorders

Name:	
Date:	
Course:	
Instructor:	

AUDIO CASE STUDY

Listen to the audio case study available on Davis Edge and then answer the following questions.

Mr. Lisle Has a Spinal Cord Injury

1. What level of spinal injury would render Jack quadriplegic?

_____

_____

2. Why is it important for Jack to direct his own care?

_____

_____

_____

3. What complications is Jack at risk for due to his quadriplegia?

_____

_____

_____

_____

4. How can you be vigilant for complications in quadriplegic patients?

Skin: _____

_____

_____

Infection: _____

_____

_____

Renal: _____

_____

_____

Autonomic dysreflexia: _____

_____

_____

VOCABULARY

Match the term with the correct definition.

1. _____ Contralateral hemiparesis
2. _____ Ipsilateral hemiplegia
3. _____ Quadriplegia
4. _____ Paraplegia
5. _____ Photophobia
6. _____ Bradykinesia
7. _____ Craniotomy
8. _____ Encephalitis
9. _____ Nuchal rigidity
10. _____ Prodromal

1. All four extremities paralyzed
2. Sensitive to light
3. Inflammation of the brain
4. Slow movement
5. Surgical opening in the skull
6. Paralyzed on same side
7. Paralyzed lower extremities
8. Neck pain and stiffness
9. Weak on opposite side
10. Warning sign

DRUGS USED FOR CENTRAL NERVOUS SYSTEM DISORDERS

Match the drug with its action.

1. _____ mannitol (Osmitrol)
2. _____ tacrine (Cognex)
3. _____ carbamazepine (Tegretol)
4. _____ dexamethasone (Decadron)
5. _____ levodopa/carbidopa (Sinemet)

1. Anticonvulsant
2. Osmotic diuretic
3. Cholinesterase inhibitor
4. Dopamine agonist that converts to dopamine in the brain
5. Corticosteroid

CENTRAL NERVOUS SYSTEM DISORDERS

Match the signs and symptoms at the left with the correct disorders at the right.

1. _____ Unconscious at accident scene
2. _____ Polyuria and polydipsia following head injury
3. _____ Hypotension and loss of sympathetic function
4. _____ Nuchal rigidity
5. _____ High blood pressure, bradycardia, and diaphoresis
6. _____ Brief period of staring
7. _____ Automatic repetitive movement such as picking or lip smacking
8. _____ Status epilepticus
9. _____ Cushing triad
10. _____ Cerebral vasoconstriction followed by vasodilation

1. Spinal shock
2. Absence seizure
3. Migraine
4. Increased intracranial pressure (ICP)
5. Meningitis
6. Diabetes insipidus
7. Autonomic dysreflexia
8. Complex partial seizure
9. Epidural bleed
10. Continuous seizure

SPINAL DISORDERS

Determine whether each of the following symptoms is associated with lumbar spine or cervical spine dysfunction. Indicate L for lumbar and C for cervical.

1. _____ Radiating pain to the ankle
2. _____ Deltoid weakness
3. _____ Diminished triceps reflex
4. _____ Foot drop
5. _____ Inability to walk on the toes

ALZHEIMER DISEASE REVIEW

Match the stage of disease with its primary symptom.

1. _____ Stage 1
2. _____ Stage 2
3. _____ Stage 3

1. Wandering, incontinence
2. Confused
3. Forgetful

CRITICAL THINKING: SPINAL CORD INJURY

Mr. Granger is a 23-year-old admitted to your unit with a C5–C6 spinal cord injury after a motor vehicle collision. You collect the following data:

Subjective Data

• Pain in cervical spine
• No sensation below the level of the injury

Objective Data

• No movement below the level of the injury
• Blood pressure 80/60 mm Hg
• Pulse 45 beats per minute
• Respirations shallow
• Temperature 97°F (36.1°C)

1. Explain Mr. Granger's hypotension, hypothermia, and bradycardia.

_____

_____

_____

_____

_____

_____

2. Why are Mr. Granger's respirations shallow?

_____

_____

_____

3. Explain the purpose of each of the following therapies. How will they benefit Mr. Granger?

   a. Cervical traction: _____

   _____

   _____

   b. Vasopressor administration: _____

   _____

   _____

   _____

   c. Insertion of a urinary catheter: _____

   _____

   _____

   _____

4. Mr. Granger suddenly becomes anxious and dyspneic. He is using his accessory muscles with each breath. Explain what might be happening.

   _____

   _____

   _____

   _____

   _____

   _____

5. What treatment would you expect for the dyspnea, and why will it be beneficial to Mr. Granger?

   _____

   _____

   _____

   _____

   _____

6. List two priority nursing diagnoses and goals for the acute stage of Mr. Granger's injury.

   _____

   _____

   _____

   _____

   _____

   _____

   _____

   _____

   _____

   _____

7. What are two health learning needs Mr. Granger faces in his acute stage?

   _____

   _____

   _____

   _____

   _____

   _____

REVIEW QUESTIONS—CONTENT REVIEW

Choose the best answer unless directed otherwise.

1. Which of the following settings is most therapeutic for an agitated patient with a head injury?
   1. A day room with family visitors and a variety of caregivers
   2. A semiprivate room with one or two consistent caregivers
   3. A ward with other patients who have head injuries and volunteers to assist with needs
   4. A hallway near the nurse's station with adequate sensory stimulation

2. Decreasing level of consciousness is a symptom of which of the following physiological phenomena?
   1. Increased intracranial pressure
   2. Sympathetic response
   3. Parasympathetic response
   4. Increased cerebral blood flow

3. Which of the following blood pressure changes alerts the nurse to increasing intracranial pressure and should be reported immediately?
   1. Gradual increase
   2. Rapid drop
   3. Widening pulse pressure
   4. Rapid fluctuations

4. Which of the following nursing interventions will help prevent a further increase in intracranial pressure?
   1. Encourage fluids.
   2. Elevate the head of the bed.
   3. Provide physical therapy.
   4. Reposition the patient frequently.

REVIEW QUESTIONS—TEST PREPARATION

Choose the best answer unless directed otherwise.

5. A 90-year-old nursing home resident with stage 2 Alzheimer disease is found alone and crying in the dining room. She says she lost her mother and doesn't know what to do. Which response by the nurse will help calm the resident?
   1. "Remember your mother has been dead for 30 years. You forgot again, didn't you?"
   2. "I'm sorry you lost your mother. Let's go and try to find her."
   3. "Are you feeling frightened? I'm here and I will help you."
   4. "You are 90 years old. It is impossible for your mother to still be living."

6. A nurse caring for a patient with a herniated lumbar disk develops a plan of care for impaired mobility related to nerve compression. Which patient outcome indicates that the plan has been successful?
   1. The patient rates the pain at 3 to 4 on a 0 to 10 scale.
   2. The patient has full range of motion of the upper extremities.
   3. The patient verbalizes the need for daily strengthening exercises.
   4. The patient is able to ambulate 25 feet safely.

7. Which of the following problems during the immediate postoperative course following lumbar microdiskectomy should be reported to the physician immediately?
   1. Incisional pain
   2. Two-inch area of bleeding on dressing
   3. Inability to move affected leg
   4. Muscle spasm of affected leg

8. A patient with a brain tumor is admitted to the medical unit to begin radiation treatments. Which nursing action should take priority?
   1. Pad the patient's side rails.
   2. Assess the patient's pain level.
   3. Teach the patient what to expect during radiation treatments.
   4. Place the patient in isolation.

9. Which nursing interventions can help prevent falls in a patient with Parkinson disease? **Select all that apply.**
   1. Keep the patient's call light within reach.
   2. Apply a soft vest restraint when the patient is in bed.
   3. Avoid use of throw rugs.
   4. Maintain the patient's bed in a low position.
   5. Encourage the patient to be independent for as long as possible.
   6. Provide a cane or walker for ambulation.

10. The nurse is counseling a young woman with a spinal cord injury at C7. Which of the following birth control options would the nurse recommend for this client? **Select all that apply.**
    1. Condom
    2. Oral contraceptives
    3. Diaphragm
    4. Implantable device
    5. Intrauterine device
    6. No birth control is needed because she will be infertile.

11. The nurse is assessing a patient admitted to a long-term care facility following a motor vehicle accident. The patient is unable to breathe without a ventilator. Mark the levels of the spinal cord that are most likely involved.

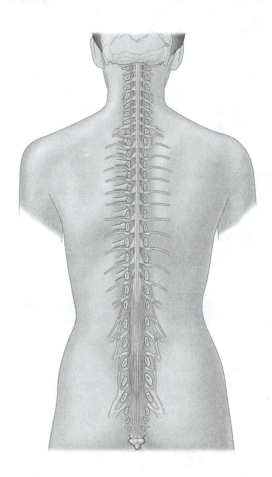

CHAPTER 49
Nursing Care of Patients With Cerebrovascular Disorders

Name:
Date:
Course:
Instructor:

AUDIO CASE STUDY

Listen to the audio case study available on Davis Edge and then answer the following questions.

Grandpa Max Has a Stroke

1. What symptoms of stroke did Amanda's grandpa exhibit? What are other signs of stroke to be aware of?

   _____

   _____

   _____

   _____

2. What does the acronym FAST stand for?

   _____

   _____

3. Why couldn't Max receive tissue plasminogen activator (tPA)?

   _____

   _____

   _____

4. What health care team members were involved in Max's care?

   _____

   _____

   _____

VOCABULARY

Match the term with the correct definition.

1. _____ Thrombotic
2. _____ Aphasia
3. _____ Dysphagia
4. _____ Hemianopsia
5. _____ Flaccid
6. _____ Ataxia
7. _____ Diplopia
8. _____ Hemiplegia
9. _____ Penumbra
10. _____ Ischemic

1. Difficulty swallowing
2. Deficient blood flow to organ or tissue
3. Inability to speak or understand language
4. Vision lost in half of visual field
5. Without muscle tone
6. Imbalanced, staggering gait
7. Caused by a clot
8. Healthy tissue surrounding an infarct
9. Double vision
10. Paralyzed on one side of the body

DRUGS USED FOR CEREBROVASCULAR DISORDERS

Match the drug with its action.

1. _____ Heparin
2. _____ Clopidogrel (Plavix)
3. _____ Tissue plasminogen activator (tPA)
4. _____ Simvastatin (Zocor)

1. Anticoagulant
2. Cholesterol-lowering agent
3. Antiplatelet
4. Thrombolytic

CRITICAL THINKING: STROKE

Read the following case study and answer the questions.

Mrs. Saunders is a 70-year-old retired secretary admitted to your unit from the emergency department with a diagnosis of stroke (cerebrovascular accident, or CVA). She has a history of hypertension and atherosclerosis, and she had a carotid endarterectomy 6 years ago. She is 40% over her ideal body weight and has a 20-pack-year smoking history. Her daughter says her mother has been having short episodes of confusion and memory loss for the past few weeks. This morning she found her mother slumped to the right in her recliner, unable to speak.

1. Explain the pathophysiology of a stroke. Which type of stroke is most likely the cause of Mrs. Saunders's symptoms?

   _____

   _____

   _____

   _____

2. Mrs. Saunders is flaccid on her right side. What is the term used to describe this?

   _____

   _____

3. Which hemisphere of Mrs. Saunders's brain is damaged?

   _____

   _____

4. List four risk factors for stroke evident in Mrs. Saunders's history.

   _____

   _____

   _____

5. Mrs. Saunders appears to understand when you speak to her but is unable to speak intelligibly. She says "plate" when she means shower and "broccoli" when she means gown. What is the term for this?

   _____

   _____

6. Neurologic checks are ordered every 2 hours for 4 hours and then every 4 hours for 4 days. When you enter her room and call her name, she opens her eyes. She is able to squeeze your hand with her left hand. However, she is only able to make incomprehensible sounds. What is her score on the Glasgow Coma Scale?

_____

_____

7. List at least three early symptoms of increasing intracranial pressure for which you will be vigilant. (You may want to refer back to Chapter 48.)

_____

_____

_____

_____

_____

8. List two medications that the health care provider may order. Why might they be used?

_____

_____

_____

_____

_____

9. Identify a nursing diagnosis related to Mrs. Saunders's right-sided paralysis. List three interventions to prevent complications.

_____

_____

_____

_____

_____

_____

10. How will you protect Mrs. Saunders's skin? List at least three interventions.

_____

_____

_____

_____

11. As you enter Mrs. Saunders's room on her third day on your unit, you find her agitated, trying to speak, and trying to get out of bed. List at least three ways to try to find out what she wants.

_____

_____

_____

_____

_____

_____

12. What should you do before feeding Mrs. Saunders for the first time?

_____

_____

_____

13. Mrs. Saunders has some difficulty swallowing and pockets her food in her right cheek. List three interventions you can try.

_____

_____

_____

_____

_____

_____

14. Mrs. Saunders begins to move her right hand slightly and is able to say her daughter's name when she enters the room. She is prepared for discharge to a rehabilitation facility. List three ways you can prepare her family for her move and her eventual discharge home.

_____

_____

_____

_____

_____

_____

_____

15. What class of drugs might be ordered for Mrs. Saunders to prevent another stroke?

_____

_____

_____

REVIEW QUESTIONS—CONTENT REVIEW

Choose the best answer unless directed otherwise.

1. What is the term or acronym for a temporary impairment of cerebral circulation that causes symptoms lasting minutes to hours but results in no permanent neurologic changes?
   1. TIA
   2. CVA
   3. SAH
   4. Stroke

2. A post–myocardial infarction patient experiencing atrial fibrillation is most at risk for which type of stroke?
   1. Hemorrhagic stroke
   2. Embolic stroke
   3. Thrombotic stroke
   4. Cerebral aneurysm

REVIEW QUESTIONS—TEST PREPARATION

Choose the best answer unless directed otherwise.

3. A nurse approaches a hospitalized post-stroke patient from the patient's left side to provide morning care. The patient is staring straight ahead and does not respond to the nurse's presence or voice. Which action should the nurse take first?
   1. Walk to the other side of the bed and try again.
   2. Speak more loudly and clearly.
   3. Wave a hand in front of the patient's face.
   4. Use a picture board to explain to the patient what the nurse is going to do.

4. A 72-year-old man is admitted to a skilled care facility following a stroke. When the nursing assistant is bathing him, he makes a sexual remark and tries to touch her inappropriately. The assistant finishes the bath and then says to the licensed practical nurse in charge, "I refuse to take care of that dirty old man!" Which response by the nurse is best?
   1. "The next time he tries to touch you inappropriately, lightly smack his hand and tell him NO!"
   2. "His stroke has made him less inhibited. We'll see if we can find a male assistant to help him."
   3. "We have to take care of all patients equally, even the dirty old men."
   4. "He didn't mean anything by it; just ignore it."

5. A patient is having difficulty swallowing following a stroke, and a swallowing evaluation is ordered. Which nursing interventions might be recommended to help prevent aspiration during eating? **Select all that apply.**
   1. Place the patient in a semi-Fowler position.
   2. Encourage the use of a straw for liquids.
   3. Provide clear liquids only until the patient can swallow solid foods.
   4. Have the patient swallow twice after each bite.
   5. Place food on the unaffected side of the patient's mouth.
   6. Check the patient's mouth for pocketing of food.

6. A patient is unable to control his bowels after a subarachnoid hemorrhage. Which intervention by the nurse can help reduce episodes of bowel incontinence?
   1. Ask the patient frequently if he has to have a bowel movement.
   2. Place incontinence pads on the patient's bed and chair.
   3. Toilet the patient according to his pre-illness schedule, whether or not he feels the urge.
   4. Take care not to embarrass the patient when incontinent episodes occur.

7. The nurse needs to administer aspirin 62 mg to a post-stroke patient. It is supplied in 1-grain tablets. How many tablets should the nurse prepare?

   _____

8. A patient is hospitalized following a stroke. Three days after admission, the patient is able to converse clearly with the nurse in the morning. Early in the afternoon, the patient's daughter runs out of the room and says, "My mother can't talk. Somebody help!" Which response by the nurse is best?
   1. Explain to the daughter that this is not uncommon, especially in the afternoon when the patient is tired from morning care activities.
   2. Do a quick assessment to confirm the change in the patient's status and then notify the registered nurse or physician immediately.
   3. Calm the daughter and then call the speech therapist to come and do a comprehensive speech assessment.
   4. Show the daughter how to help her mother do the speech exercises that were provided by the therapist.

9. The nurse is caring for a patient recently admitted with a stroke. The patient is experiencing nausea and begins to vomit. Which of the following actions should the nurse take first?
   1. Call for an aide to get suction set up.
   2. Assist the patient to turn to his side.
   3. Give an antiemetic as ordered.
   4. Perform a test for blood on the emesis.

10. The nurse is providing care for a patient with a hemorrhagic stroke. Which of the following medication orders would the nurse question? **Select all that apply.**
    1. Simvastatin (Zocor)
    2. Clopidogrel (Plavix)
    3. Carbamazepine (Tegretol)
    4. Tissue plasminogen activator (tPA)
    5. Metoprolol (Toprol)
    6. Warfarin (Coumadin)

11. A 67-year-old gentleman being evaluated and treated in the emergency department for a stroke has clopidogrel (Plavix) ordered per os (PO) now. Which of the following would cause the nurse to hold the medication? **Select all that apply.**
    1. The patient has weak grip strength in the right hand and strong in the left.
    2. The patient's smile is crooked.
    3. The patient's gag reflex is positive.
    4. The patient's voice sounds gurgly after taking a sip of water.
    5. The patient's blood pressure is 168/90 mm Hg.
    6. The patient has an allergy to aspirin.

CHAPTER 50

Nursing Care of Patients With Peripheral Nervous System Disorders

Name:	
Date:	
Course:	
Instructor:	

AUDIO CASE STUDY

Listen to the audio case study available on Davis Edge and then answer the following questions.

Mrs. Mead Has Myasthenia Gravis

1. Why are the eyes often affected first in myasthenia gravis?

_____

_____

2. In what drug class is edrophonium (Tensilon)? What happens when it is injected?

_____

_____

_____

3. What are three things that should be taught to all patients with myasthenia gravis?

_____

_____

_____

_____

_____

_____

VOCABULARY

Fill in the blanks with the correct terms.

1. Muscles that are not used become wasted, or _____.
2. Some diseases are characterized by remissions and _____.
3. Nerve pain is also called _____.
4. An early symptom of myasthenia gravis is drooping eyelids, also called _____.
5. Symptoms of Guillain-Barré syndrome are caused by _____ of axons.
6. Myasthenia gravis is sometimes treated with _____, which separates blood cells from plasma to remove antibodies.
7. Muscle twitching, or _____, occurs in amyotrophic lateral sclerosis.
8. Medications for myasthenia gravis that can increase acetylcholine at the neuromuscular junction are called _____ agents.

PERIPHERAL NERVOUS SYSTEM DISORDERS

Underline incorrect information in the following case studies. Write the correct information in the space provided.

1. Ms. Mary Garvey sees her physician because she has been seeing double off and on for several weeks and has been fatigued. Her physician suspects myasthenia gravis and schedules her for a carotid ultrasound. He confirms his suspicions with a Tensilon (edrophonium) test. He explains to Ms. Garvey that she has a disease that is characterized by a decrease in the neurotransmitter norepinephrine. He begins her on Mastodon and prednisone. Her nurse teaches her the importance of getting regular exercise and recommends joining a local health and exercise club.

   _____
   _____
   _____

2. Mr. Tom Newby has a history of trigeminal neuralgia. He enters the emergency department with severe pain in his left wrist. The physician orders a narcotic analgesic because Mr. Newby's third cranial nerve is inflamed. Once the acute pain has subsided, Mr. Newby is discharged with instructions to get plenty of fresh air and to take his gabapentin (Neurontin) as ordered.

   _____
   _____
   _____

3. Mrs. Mattie Schultz is admitted with exacerbated multiple sclerosis (MS). Her legs are becoming weaker, causing difficulty walking, and she has been having difficulty swallowing. You know that buildup of myelin on her neurons is responsible for her weakness. You assess her for stressors that might have caused her exacerbation, such as a urinary tract infection (UTI) or upper respiratory tract infection. Mrs. Schultz is started on thyroid-stimulating hormone (TSH) to stimulate her thyroid, which will help reduce her symptoms. She is also placed on trimethoprim/sulfamethoxazole (Bactrim) for the UTI you identified through your excellent assessment and on diazepam (Valium) for urinary retention.

   _____
   _____
   _____

CRITICAL THINKING

Read the following case study and answer the questions.

Reverend Wilson is a 50-year-old minister who sees his physician when he develops weakness in his arms and legs and has difficulty carrying out his job duties. He is diagnosed with amyotrophic lateral sclerosis (ALS).

1. Reverend Wilson's wife asks what ALS is. How do you describe it to her?

   _____

   _____

   _____

2. Reverend Wilson returns to the physician's office several months after his initial diagnosis because he fell walking to the podium to preach. What is happening? What can he do about it?

   _____

   _____

   _____

3. Reverend Wilson is concerned about continuing in his job and asks if his mind is going to be affected. How do you respond?

   _____

   _____

   _____

4. He develops painful muscle spasms. What medications might be ordered to help relieve them?

   _____

   _____

   _____

5. Reverend Wilson stabilizes for a while. A year later, he is admitted to the hospital with aspiration pneumonia. What probably happened? What nursing diagnosis is appropriate in this situation? List an appropriate goal and two or three interventions.

   _____

   _____

   _____

6. Reverend Wilson's condition deteriorates, and he has to retire. He becomes confined to a wheelchair. He has a gastrostomy tube inserted because he is no longer able to swallow. What additional nursing diagnoses are now appropriate?

   _____

   _____

   _____

REVIEW QUESTIONS—CONTENT REVIEW

Choose the best answer unless directed otherwise.

1. Which medication class is used to reduce symptoms of muscle weakness from myasthenia gravis?
   1. Anticholinesterase
   2. Anticholinergic
   3. Adrenergic
   4. Beta blocker

2. Which of the following nursing interventions will help prevent complications in the patient with Bell palsy?
   1. Vitamin therapy
   2. Elastic bandages
   3. Application of ice to the affected area
   4. Lubricating eyedrops

3. Which data collection activity will help the nurse determine if the patient with Bell palsy is receiving adequate nutrition?
   1. Monitor meal trays.
   2. Measure intake and output.
   3. Check twice-weekly weights.
   4. Evaluate swallowing reflex.

REVIEW QUESTIONS—TEST PREPARATION

Choose the best answer unless directed otherwise.

4. A patient is admitted to a medical unit with a diagnosis of Guillain-Barré syndrome. The patient's legs are weak, causing difficulty walking without assistance. Which of the following is most likely responsible for this syndrome?
   1. Bacterial infection
   2. Heredity
   3. High-fat diet
   4. Autoimmune reaction

5. Patients with Guillain-Barré syndrome should be closely monitored. Which of the following lab results is most important to monitor for acute complications?
   1. Blood urea nitrogen and creatinine
   2. Arterial blood gases
   3. Hemoglobin and hematocrit
   4. Serum potassium

6. A patient sees a health care provider because of extreme fatigue for 2 months and difficulty lifting even light objects. The health care provider suspects myasthenia gravis. Which of the following tests should the nurse anticipate assisting with to confirm this diagnosis?
   1. Mestinon (pyridostigmine) test
   2. Quinine tolerance test
   3. Pulmonary function studies
   4. Tensilon (edrophonium) test

7. A patient sees the health care provider after falling twice for seemingly no reason. Diagnostic tests are done, and the patient is diagnosed with multiple sclerosis. Which of the following explanations will help the patient understand the disease?
   1. "You have a buildup of myelin in your nervous system, causing congestion and muscle weakness."
   2. "You are missing a neurotransmitter that is important to muscle contraction."
   3. "The receptor sites on your muscles are damaged, so they can't contract correctly."
   4. "The insulation on your nerve cells is damaged, which slows the impulses to the muscles."

8. A patient newly diagnosed with amyotrophic lateral sclerosis verbalizes not wanting to be "kept alive on machines." Which response by the nurse is most appropriate?
   1. "I'm sorry to hear that. Your family might feel differently."
   2. "Do you have your advance directive prepared?"
   3. "I will request a hospice referral for you."
   4. "It is too early to make such decisions. Don't think about it yet."

9. A home health care nurse is developing a plan of care designed to prevent complications in a patient with impaired respiratory function secondary to a neurological disorder. Which of the following would the nurse include in the plan? **Select all that apply.**
   1. Monitor oxygen saturation and respiratory rate and depth.
   2. Elevate the head of the bed.
   3. Maintain patient on bedrest.
   4. Suction every 4 hours.
   5. Encourage patient to deep breathe and cough every 2 hours.

10. A nurse is preparing an intramuscular injection of prednisolone acetate, 30 mg. It is supplied as 50 mg/mL. How many milliliters should the nurse prepare? _____

11. The nurse notes frequent muscle twitching when collecting admission data on a patient admitted for increasing muscle weakness. Which of the following terms should be used to document this?
    1. Fasciculation
    2. Atrophy
    3. Chorea
    4. Neuropathy

12. A 19-year-old student develops trigeminal neuralgia. Which of the following actions is most likely to trigger pain?
    1. Sleeping
    2. Eating
    3. Reading
    4. Cooking

CHAPTER 51

Sensory System Function, Assessment, and Therapeutic Measures: Vision and Hearing

Name: _____	
Date: _____	
Course: _____	
Instructor: _____	

AUDIO CASE STUDY

Listen to the audio case study available on Davis Edge and then answer the following questions.

Selena and Sensory Care

1. How should one enter the room of a person who is blind?

   _____

   _____

2. How can vision and safety be enhanced for glasses wearers?

   _____

   _____

   _____

3. Why did Selena take the time to obtain the hearing aid for Ted?

   _____

   _____

4. How are eye drops given to a patient?

_____

_____

_____

_____

_____

_____

STRUCTURES OF THE EYE

Label the following structures.

Anterior chamber

Aqueous humor

Canal of Schlemm

Choroid layer

Ciliary body

Conjunctiva

Cornea

Fovea

Inferior rectus muscle

Iris

Lens

Optic disc

Optic nerve

Posterior chamber

Pupil

Retina

Retinal artery and vein

Sclera

Vitreous humor

Superior rectus muscle

Suspensory ligaments

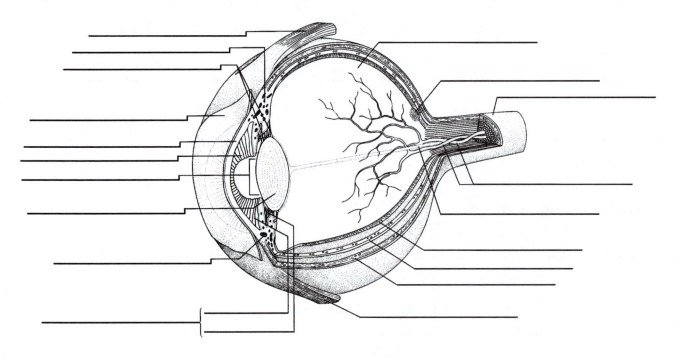

STRUCTURES OF THE EAR

Label the following structures.

Auricle   Malleus
Cochlea   Semicircular canals
Cochlear nerve (8th)   Stapes
Ear canal   Tympanic membrane (eardrum)
Eustachian tube   Utricle and saccule
Incus   Vestibular nerve (8th)

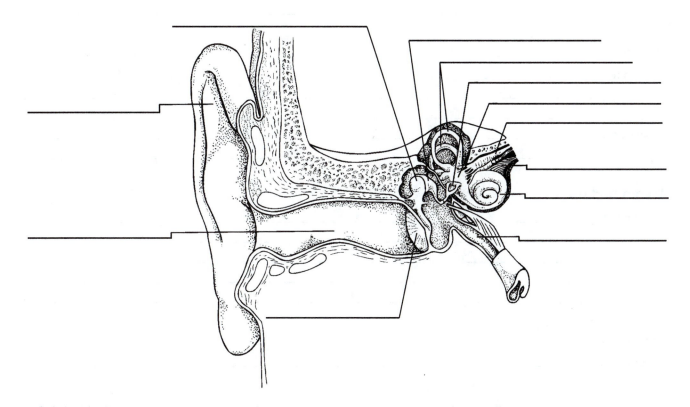

VISION

Number the following in the proper sequence as they are involved in the process of producing a visual image from the beginning to end.

_____ A. Cornea   _____ E. Occipital lobe
_____ B. Vitreous humor   _____ F. Lens
_____ C. Optic nerve   _____ G. Retina
_____ D. Aqueous humor

HEARING

Number the following in the order they function in the process of hearing when sound waves enter the ear canal.

_____ A. Eardrum   _____ F. Stapes
_____ B. Oval window   _____ G. Fluid in the cochlea
_____ C. Incus   _____ H. Hair cells in the organ of Corti
_____ D. Eighth cranial nerve   _____ I. Temporal lobes
_____ E. Malleus

VOCABULARY

Define the following terms and use them in a sentence.

Nystagmus

Definition: _____

_____

_____

Sentence: _____

_____

Tropia

Definition: _____

_____

_____

Sentence: _____

_____

Accommodation

Definition: _____

_____

_____

Sentence: _____

_____

Ptosis

Definition: _____

_____

_____

Sentence: _____

_____

Arcus senilis

Definition: _____

_____

_____

Sentence: _____

_____

Ophthalmologist

Definition: _____

_____

_____

Sentence: _____

_____

Optometrist

Definition: _____

_____

_____

Sentence: _____

_____

Optician

Definition: _____

_____

_____

Sentence: _____

_____

DIAGNOSTIC TESTS

Fill in the table.

Assessment Test	Purpose of Test	Normal Test Results
Snellen chart Visual fields	_____ _____ _____	Right eye (OD) 20/20, Left eye (OS) 20/20 _____ _____
Cardinal fields of gaze	Extraocular movement	_____ _____ _____
Accommodation	_____ _____	Eyes turn inward and pupils constrict when focusing on a near object
Rinne	_____ _____ _____	Air conduction greater than bone conduction.
Weber	_____ _____	_____
Romberg	Balance/vestibular function	_____ _____ _____

CRITICAL THINKING

Read the following case study and answer the questions.

Ms. Litley works on a computer as a data processor. She reports that she has recurring eye discomfort about 2 hours after she begins work each day.

1. What might the nurse suspect is occurring with Ms. Litley?

   _____

   _____

2. For what environmental factors should the nurse gather data?

   _____

   _____

3. To protect Ms. Litley from eye strain, what safety measures should be implemented in her office?

   _____

   _____

   _____

   _____

   _____

   _____

REVIEW QUESTIONS—CONTENT REVIEW

Choose the best answer unless directed otherwise.

1. If documented in the patient's history, which physical examination finding would indicate that the patient has a normal corneal light reflex?
   1. The eye focuses the image in the center of the pupil.
   2. The eyes converge to focus on the light.
   3. Constriction of both pupils occurs in response to bright light.
   4. Light is reflected at the same spot in both eyes.

2. When testing visual fields, the nurse examines which part of vision?
   1. Peripheral vision
   2. Near vision
   3. Distance vision
   4. Central vision

3. Which term would indicate to the nurse that a substance is toxic to the ear?
   1. Otoplasty
   2. Otalgia
   3. Ototoxic
   4. Tinnitus

4. Which test would the nurse use as an initial screening test to determine hearing loss?
   1. Romberg test
   2. Otoscopic examination
   3. Caloric test
   4. Whisper voice test

5. Which term would the nurse use to document a finding that the patient's ear is draining?
   1. Otorrhea
   2. Otalgia
   3. Ototoxic
   4. Tinnitus

6. Which term indicates that the patient has hearing loss caused by aging?
   1. Otoplasty
   2. Otalgia
   3. Presbycusis
   4. Tinnitus

REVIEW QUESTIONS—TEST PREPARATION

Choose the best answer unless directed otherwise.

7. Which explanation would the nurse give to the patient who had a Snellen chart finding of 20/80?
   1. "You can see at 80 feet what those with normal vision can see at 20 feet."
   2. "You can see at 20 feet what those with normal vision can see at 80 feet."
   3. "You can see four times farther than those with normal vision can see."
   4. "Your vision is normal."

8. The nurse shines a penlight in the patient's eyes and finds the pupils are round and constrict from 4 to 2 mm bilaterally. Next, the nurse asks the patient to focus on a far object, then on the nurse's finger as it is brought in from a distance of 3 feet to 5 inches. The pupils constrict bilaterally, and the eyes turn inward. Which would be the correct documentation of these findings?
   1. Pupils 2 mm
   2. Pupils constricted
   3. Pupils equal, round, and reactive to light and accommodation (PERRLA)
   4. Pupils normal

9. In planning safe care for the older adult, which of these conditions does the nurse recognize would cause visual problems? **Select all that apply.**
   1. Glaucoma
   2. Cataracts
   3. Arcus senilis
   4. Macular degeneration
   5. Esotropia
   6. Presbycusis

10. Which finding would the nurse understand is normal when checking auditory acuity using the Rinne test?
    1. The patient perceives sound equally in both ears.
    2. Air conduction is heard longer than bone conduction in both ears.
    3. Bone conduction is heard longer than air conduction in both ears.
    4. The patient's left ear will perceive the sound better than the right ear.

11. Which data collection finding could indicate to the nurse that the patient has a hearing loss? **Select all that apply.**
    1. Patient converses easily with nurse.
    2. Patient answers questions appropriately.
    3. Patient's face is relaxed during conversation.
    4. Patient speaks in a very loud voice.
    5. Patient turns toward person speaking.
    6. Patient is withdrawn.

12. Which subjective data question should the nurse ask while collecting data about the patient's eye health?
    1. "Have you had any recent upper respiratory infections?"
    2. "Have you been on an airplane recently?"
    3. "Have you been scuba diving lately?"
    4. "Have you seen halos around lights?"

13. When collecting data on a patient's external ear, the nurse palpates a small protrusion of the helix called the Darwin tubercle. What action would the nurse take for this finding?
    1. Document it, as it is a normal finding.
    2. Report it to the registered nurse, as it is an abnormal finding.
    3. Report it to the health care provider immediately, as it is a serious finding.
    4. Inform the patient that further testing for this finding will need to be ordered.

14. The nurse is to administer eye drops. Mark the area where the nurse should apply pressure after administering the eye drops.

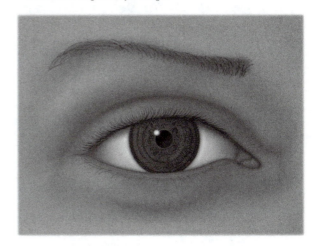

CHAPTER 52

Nursing Care of Patients With Sensory Disorders: Vision and Hearing

Name:	_____
Date:	_____
Course:	_____
Instructor:	_____

AUDIO CASE STUDY

Listen to the audio case study available on Davis Edge and then answer the following questions.

Sally and Ménière Disease

1. What effect of Ménière disease did Jan experience that can be a safety concern?

   _____

   _____

2. What symptoms of Ménière disease did Jan experience?

   _____

   _____

3. What is a safety concern for those with Ménière disease?

   _____

   _____

4. What medications are used for Ménière disease?

   _____

   _____

VOCABULARY

Match the following terms with their appropriate definitions.

1. _____ Carbuncle
2. _____ Cholesteatoma
3. _____ Mastoiditis
4. _____ Barotrauma
5. _____ Labyrinthitis
6. _____ Presbycusis

1. Hearing loss caused by aging
2. Inflammation or infection of the inner ear
3. Complication of otitis media
4. Epithelial cystlike sac filled with skin and sebaceous material
5. Several hair follicles forming an abscess
6. Pressure in the middle ear caused by atmospheric changes

ERRORS OF REFRACTION

Draw pictures showing the eye size and focal point differences in (a) hyperopia and (b) myopia.

VISUAL AND HEARING DATA COLLECTION

List findings that would be present during data collection for the following conditions, including signs and symptoms, diagnostic tests, and physical examinations.

Macular degeneration (dry type) _____

_____

_____

_____

_____

_____

Cataract _____

_____

_____

_____

_____

_____

Hordeolum _____

_____

Acute angle-closure glaucoma _____

_____

_____

_____

External otitis _____

_____

_____

Impacted cerumen _____

_____

_____

_____

Otitis media _____

_____

_____

_____

Otosclerosis _____

_____

_____

_____

_____

_____

_____

PRESBYOPIA

Circle the seven errors in the following paragraph and insert the correct information.

Presbyopia is a condition in which the lenses increase their elasticity, resulting in a decrease in ability to focus on far objects. The loss of elasticity causes light rays to focus in front of the retina, resulting in hyperopia. This condition is usually associated with aging and generally occurs before age 40. Because accommodation for close vision is accomplished by lens contraction, people with presbyopia exhibit the ability to see objects at close range. They often compensate for blurred close vision by holding objects to be viewed closer. Complaints of eye strain and mild occipital headache are common.

GLAUCOMA

Circle the seven errors in the following paragraph and insert the correct information.

Glaucoma may be characterized by abnormal pressure outside the eyeball. This pressure causes damage to the cells of the acoustic nerve, the structure responsible for transmitting visual information from the ear to the brain. The damage is evident, progressive, and reversible until the end stage, when loss of central vision occurs and eventually blindness. Once glaucoma occurs, the patient can be cured.

CONDUCTIVE HEARING LOSS

Circle the seven errors in the following paragraph and insert the correct information.

Conductive hearing loss is interference with conduction of light waves through the external auditory canal, eardrum, or middle ear. The inner ear is involved in a pure conductive hearing loss. Conductive hearing loss is a neural problem. Causes of conductive hearing loss include cerumen, foreign bodies, infection, perforation of the tympanic membrane, trauma, fluid in the inner ear, cysts, tumor, and otosclerosis. Many causes of conductive hearing loss, such as infection, foreign bodies, or impacted cerumen, cannot be corrected. Hearing devices may not improve hearing for conditions that cannot be corrected. Hearing devices are most effective with conductive hearing loss when inner ear and nerve damage are present.

OTOSCLEROSIS

Circle the nine errors in the following paragraph and insert the correct information.

Otosclerosis results from the formation of new bone along the incus. With new bone growth, the incus becomes mobile, which causes conductive hearing loss. Hearing loss is most apparent after the sixth decade. Otosclerosis usually occurs less frequently in women than in men. The disease usually affects one ear. It is thought to be a hereditary disease. The primary symptom of otosclerosis is rapid hearing loss. The patient usually experiences bilateral conductive hearing loss, particularly with soft, high tones. Otectomy is the treatment of choice.

CRITICAL THINKING

Read the following case study and answer the questions.

Mr. Nyugen, age 70, reports that he has difficulty seeing at night and has given up driving. When questioned further, he also states, "I used to be an avid reader, but I guess I'm getting too old to read. The words aren't very clear." The nurse checks his eyes and finds that he is sensitive to light, has opacity of both lenses, and has no pain. The nurse informs the health care provider of these findings who plans further testing.

1. What might the nurse suspect is occurring with Mr. Nyugen?

   _____

   _____

   _____

   _____

2. For which diagnostic tests should the nurse prepare Mr. Nyugen?

   _____

   _____

   _____

   _____

   _____

   _____

3. After the health care provider has made a definitive diagnosis of cataracts, the nurse develops a teaching plan. What should the nurse include in the teaching plan?

   _____

   _____

   _____

   _____

REVIEW QUESTIONS—CONTENT REVIEW

Choose the best answer unless directed otherwise.

1. Which type of eye drop does the nurse understand is given to constrict the pupil, permitting aqueous humor to flow around the lens?
   1. Osmotic
   2. Myotic
   3. Mydriatic
   4. Cycloplegic

2. Which procedure does the nurse understand is used to drain fluid from the inner ear?
   1. Myringotomy
   2. Myringoplasty
   3. Mastoidectomy
   4. Stapedectomy

3. The nurse understands that labyrinthitis is treated primarily with which drug category?
   1. Antihistamines
   2. Antispasmodics
   3. Anti-inflammatories
   4. Antiemetics

4. Which of the following types of hearing loss does the nurse understand is most improved with the use of a hearing aid?
   1. Conductive
   2. Sensorineural
   3. Mixed
   4. Central

5. The nurse would teach the patient that otitis media occurs in which part of the ear?
   1. Outer ear
   2. Inner ear
   3. Middle ear
   4. Semicircular canal

REVIEW QUESTIONS—TEST PREPARATION

Choose the best answer unless directed otherwise.

6. The nurse is assisting with data collection for a patient with macular degeneration. Which symptoms would the nurse expect to be present? **Select all that apply.**
   1. Decreased distinction of colors
   2. Sudden loss of vision
   3. Loss of near vision
   4. Loss of central vision
   5. Loss of peripheral vision
   6. Increased periodic dizziness

7. The nurse is caring for a patient after cataract surgery. Which safety instruction should the nurse give this patient? **Select all that apply.**
   1. Elevate the head of your bed 45 degrees.
   2. Avoid swimming after surgery.
   3. Avoid caffeinated beverages.
   4. Report sudden sharp pain to the health care provider.
   5. Report increased drainage to the health care provider.
   6. Keep follow-up appointment after surgery.

8. The nurse is assisting a patient who has recently received a hearing aid. Which response by the patient would indicate further teaching is required about the care of the hearing aid?
   1. "Turning off the hearing aid when not in use saves the battery."
   2. "The hearing aid can be washed daily in a basin of warm water."
   3. "A small brush can be used to clean in the ear mold."
   4. "I should remove the hearing aid before showering."

9. The nurse is reinforcing teaching for a patient with Ménière disease. Which of the following would the nurse explain to the patient is the triad of symptoms associated with Ménière disease? **Select all that apply.**
   1. Hearing loss
   2. Headache
   3. Nausea
   4. Tinnitus
   5. Vertigo
   6. Vomiting

10. The nurse is reinforcing teaching for the patient with vertigo. Which of the following statements by the patient for actions to take for vertigo would indicate that further teaching is needed? **Select all that apply.**
    1. "I will avoid noise."
    2. "I should avoid sudden movements."
    3. "I will increase my fluid intake."
    4. "I will take analgesics."
    5. "I will lie down for safety."
    6. "I should walk frequently."

11. In providing patient teaching for acute bacterial conjunctivitis, the nurse would evaluate the patient as understanding the teaching if the patient stated that this condition is more commonly known as which of the following?
    1. Astigmatism
    2. Color blindness
    3. Glaucoma
    4. Pink eye

12. The nurse is collecting data on a patient with a cataract. What is usually the first symptom of a cataract that the nurse would expect a patient to report?
    1. Dry eyes
    2. Eye pain
    3. Blurring of vision
    4. Loss of peripheral vision

13. The nurse is caring for a patient after eye surgery. Which nursing intervention would have the highest priority in the plan of care for the postoperative eye patient?
    1. Do not leave the patient unattended at any time.
    2. Teach the patient not to bend over.
    3. Report sudden onset of acute pain.
    4. Apply sandbags to either side of the head.

14. The nurse is teaching a patient with newly diagnosed glaucoma. The nurse would evaluate the patient as understanding the teaching if the patient stated which of these definitions for glaucoma?
    1. "The rate of production of aqueous humor decreases."
    2. "There is an increase in the pressure within the eye."
    3. "There is a decrease in the amount of aqueous humor."
    4. "There is an increase in the amount of vitreous humor."

15. The nurse is caring for a patient with acute angle-closure glaucoma. Which symptoms would the nurse expect to find during data collection for this patient? **Select all that apply.**
    1. Flashing lights
    2. Lens opacity
    3. Photophobia
    4. Rainbows around lights
    5. Severe pain over eye
    6. Steamy-appearing cornea

16. The nurse is caring for a patient after eye surgery. Which activities would the nurse teach a patient to avoid so that intraocular pressure is not increased after eye surgery? **Select all that apply.**
    1. Bending over
    2. Chewing food vigorously
    3. Coughing
    4. Reading
    5. Sitting upright in bed
    6. Sneezing

17. A patient with acute angle-closure glaucoma reports use of the following medications. The use of which of these medications indicates to the nurse that the patient requires further instruction? **Select all that apply.**
    1. Acetaminophen
    2. Atropine (Isopto Atropine)
    3. Diphenhydramine (Benadryl)
    4. Digoxin (Lanoxin)
    5. Furosemide (Lasix)
    6. Timolol (Timoptic)

18. The nurse is teaching the patient ear care after ear surgery. The nurse would evaluate the patient as understanding the teaching if the patient stated which of these ways to care for the ear after surgery?
    1. "I will blow my nose very gently for the first week after surgery."
    2. "I should blow both sides of my nose at the same time."
    3. "I will avoid sneezing for 2 weeks."
    4. "I will cough with my mouth open for 1 week after surgery."
    5. "I will not fly for 1 week after surgery."
    6. "I will change the cotton plug daily."

CHAPTER 53

Integumentary System Function, Assessment, and Therapeutic Measures

Name: _____	
Date: _____	
Course: _____	
Instructor: _____	

AUDIO CASE STUDY

Listen to the audio case study available on Davis Edge and then answer the following questions.

Hakem Assesses Skin Lesions

1. What is the difference between a vesicle and a bulla?

   _____

   _____

2. What disorder did Hakem see that had scales and plaques?

   _____

   _____

3. What term would you use to describe small, red raised areas?

   _____

   _____

4. How should ointment be applied to a wound prior to applying an occlusive dressing?

   _____

   _____

INTEGUMENTARY STRUCTURES

Match each integumentary structure with its appropriate description.

1. _____ Epidermis
2. _____ Dermis
3. _____ Subcutaneous tissue
4. _____ Collagen fibers
5. _____ Eccrine glands
6. _____ Receptors
7. _____ Melanin
8. _____ Stratum corneum
9. _____ Stratum germinativum

1. If unbroken, prevents entry of pathogens
2. Give strength to the dermis
3. Detect changes in the external environment
4. Contains the accessory structures of the skin, such as glands
5. Made of both living and nonliving cells
6. Mitosis takes place to produce new epidermis
7. Stores fat
8. Acts as a barrier to ultraviolet (UV) light
9. Stimulated by exercise or heat

VOCABULARY

Match the word at the right with its definition at the left.

1. _____ Absence or loss of hair
2. _____ Blue-black bruise, changing to greenish brown or yellow with time
3. _____ Diffuse redness over the skin
4. _____ Small, purplish, hemorrhagic spots on the skin
5. _____ Measure of skin elasticity and hydration

1. Ecchymosis
2. Erythema
3. Petechiae
4. Turgor
5. Alopecia

DIAGNOSTIC SKIN TESTS

Match the test with its definition.

1. _____ Skin biopsy
2. _____ Wood light examination
3. _____ Scratch test
4. _____ Patch test

1. Superficial testing with allergen for immediate reaction
2. Excision of a small piece of tissue for microscopic assessment
3. Superficial testing with allergen for delayed hypersensitivity reaction
4. Use of UV rays to detect fluorescent materials in skin and hair

PRIMARY SKIN LESIONS

Match the lesion with its description.

1. _____ Macule
2. _____ Papule
3. _____ Vesicle
4. _____ Bulla
5. _____ Pustule
6. _____ Wheal
7. _____ Plaque
8. _____ Cyst

1. Vesicle or blister larger than 1 cm
2. Flat, nonpalpable change in skin color
3. Round, transient elevation of the skin caused by dermal edema and surrounding capillary dilation
4. Patch or solid, raised lesion on the skin or mucous membrane that is greater than 1 cm
5. Palpable, solid raised lesion
6. Small elevation of skin or vesicle or bulla that contains pus
7. Closed sac or pouch tumor that consists of semisolid, solid, or liquid material
8. Small raised area that contains serous fluid, less than 1 cm

CRITICAL THINKING

A 90-year-old female patient is admitted to the long-term care facility where you work. Her husband, age 94, was caring for her, but he is no longer able to do so. On admission, you note that she is very thin and confused and has multiple lesions on her extremities, torso, and coccyx.

1. Identify the term to use for documenting each of the following problems.
   a. Small, fluid-filled blisters on her torso, about 0.8 cm each. _____
   b. Large open area on her coccyx, 4 cm x 6 cm, approximately 1 cm deep, from lying on her back. It is draining
      yellowish-green purulent material. _____
   c. Thin flap of skin on her arm that exposes the underlying dermis. _____
   d. Multiple large bruised areas on her arms and legs. _____
   e. Bluish cast to her lips and toes. _____

2. List options for dressings that will help the following skin problems she is experiencing, and explain why they might help.
   a. Wound on coccyx: _____
   _____
   _____
   _____

   b. Exposed dermis on arm: _____
   _____
   _____
   _____

REVIEW QUESTIONS—CONTENT REVIEW

Choose the best answer unless directed otherwise.

1. How do arterioles in the dermis respond to a cold environment?
   1. Dilate to release heat
   2. Constrict to release heat
   3. Dilate to conserve heat
   4. Constrict to conserve heat

2. Which of the following tissues stores fat in subcutaneous tissue?
   1. Fibrous connective tissue
   2. Stratified squamous epithelium
   3. Adipose tissue
   4. Areolar connective tissue

3. Which substances are formed when the ultraviolet rays of the sun strike the skin?
   1. Vitamin A and keratin
   2. Melanin and vitamin D
   3. Sebum and vitamin A
   4. Keratin and melanin

4. Which layer of skin, if unbroken, prevents the entry of most pathogens?
   1. Stratum corneum
   2. Papillary layer
   3. Stratum germinativum
   4. Dermis

5. White blood cells, which destroy pathogens that enter breaks in the skin, are found in which of the following structures?
   1. Stratum corneum
   2. Keratinized layer
   3. Subcutaneous tissue
   4. Adipose cells

6. The nurse is assessing a patient with a macular rash due to a reaction to antibiotics. Mark the image that represents a macule.

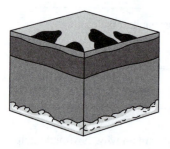 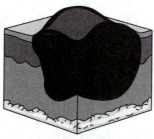 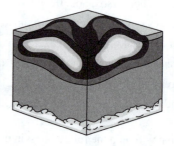 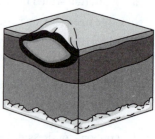

REVIEW QUESTIONS—TEST PREPARATION

7. The nurse is reviewing a patient chart and notes the following: "poor elasticity and dry, thin skin noted." The nurse recognizes this is a normal finding for which of the following patient groups?
   1. Adolescents
   2. Young adults
   3. Middle-aged adults
   4. Older adults

8. When assessing a patient in hospice who is near death, the nurse notes a bluish discoloration and mottled appearance on the patient's feet and lower legs. Which of the following terms would the nurse use to best document this finding?
   1. Cyanosis
   2. Erythema
   3. Jaundice
   4. Pallor

9. A nurse is providing care for an older adult patient who reports being sensitive to cold temperatures. The nurse would base teaching on which of the following principles?
   1. There is slower cell division in the epidermis with aging.
   2. Older adults experience deterioration of collagen and elastin fibers.
   3. There is less fat in the subcutaneous layer with age.
   4. Death of melanocytes in the skin occurs with age.

10. Which of the following dressing types is most appropriate for the nurse to apply to a skin tear in an older adult patient?
    1. Moist, sterile gauze
    2. Transparent dressing
    3. Paste
    4. Nonadherent dressing

11. Which of the following actions should the nurse take when new petechiae are observed on a patient's skin?
    1. Cleanse the skin.
    2. Apply cool compresses.
    3. Inform the registered nurse or physician.
    4. Apply heat to the area.

12. A nurse is preparing to collect a wound culture. Which of the following would be included in the collection process? **Select all that apply.**
    1. Swab wound and wound edges in a rotating motion.
    2. Swab over areas of eschar.
    3. Use sterile saline to remove excess debris before culture.
    4. Use clean cotton-tipped swab to collect purulent drainage.
    5. Swab wound 10 times in a diagonal pattern.
    6. Obtain sterile calcium alginate swab for culture collection.

CHAPTER 54
Nursing Care of Patients With Skin Disorders

Name:	
Date:	
Course:	
Instructor:	

AUDIO CASE STUDY

Mr. Fletcher's Pressure Injuries

Listen to the audio case study available on Davis Edge and then answer the following questions.

1. What risk factors for pressure injuries did Mr. Fletcher have?

   _____

   _____

2. What are characteristics of stage 1, 2, 3, and 4 pressure injuries?

   _____

   _____

   _____

   _____

   _____

   _____

   _____

   _____

   _____

   _____

3. How was Patrick vigilant in helping Mr. Fletcher heal and in preventing new pressure injuries?

   _____

   _____

   _____

VOCABULARY

Match the word with its definition.

1. _____ To lose color
2. _____ Inflammation of cellular or connective tissue
3. _____ Skin lesion that occurs in acne vulgaris
4. _____ Inflammation of the skin
5. _____ Thickened or hardened from continued irritation
6. _____ Disease of the nails due to fungus
7. _____ Infestation with lice
8. _____ Severe itching
9. _____ Chronic inflammatory skin disorder in which epidermal cells proliferate abnormally quickly
10. _____ Describes fluid that contains pus
11. _____ Any acute, inflammatory, purulent bacterial dermatitis
12. _____ Disease of the sebaceous glands marked by increase in the amount, and often alteration of the quality, of sebaceous secretion

1. Seborrhea
2. Pyoderma
3. Purulent
4. Psoriasis
5. Pruritus
6. Pediculosis
7. Onychomycosis
8. Lichenified
9. Dermatitis
10. Comedo
11. Cellulitis
12. Blanch

BENIGN SKIN LESIONS

Match the lesion with its definition.

1. _____ Cyst
2. _____ Seborrheic keratosis
3. _____ Keloid
4. _____ Pigmented nevi
5. _____ Warts
6. _____ Hemangiomas

1. Small, common growths caused by a virus
2. Vascular tumors of dilated blood vessels
3. Saclike growth with a definite wall
4. Excessive scar formation at site of trauma or surgical incision
5. Light brown to dark brown patches, plaques, or papules that occur mainly in older patients
6. Flesh-colored to dark brown macule or papule

PLASTIC SURGERY PROCEDURES

Fill in the blanks.

1. A _____ is done to correct nasal shape or septal defects.

2. A _____ is referred to as a rhytidoplasty.

3. Removal of bags under the eyes is known as _____.

CRITICAL THINKING

Read the following case study and answer the questions.

Mr. Carr is admitted to a medical unit after having a hemorrhagic stroke. His vital signs are stable, but he is disoriented except to person. He is on bed rest and is often restless. He responds appropriately to questions intermittently. His left side is flaccid, but he can move his right side. The nurse notes that Mr. Carr rarely moves himself into a different position. He is of thin build. He is receiving 5% dextrose/0.9% normal saline intravenously. He has difficulty swallowing and has not eaten. Mr. Carr is diaphoretic and his gown is damp.

1. Why is Mr. Carr at high risk for developing pressure injuries?

   _____

   _____

   _____

   _____

   _____

2. What are priority nursing diagnoses and nursing interventions for Mr. Carr related to his skin needs?

   _____

   _____

   _____

   _____

   _____

   _____

   _____

   _____

   _____

CRITICAL THINKING

Read the following case study and answer the questions.

Mrs. Miller, age 59, is admitted for a femoral-popliteal bypass graft. She has type 2 diabetes mellitus. After surgery, she is in the intensive care unit and is hypotensive for 24 hours. Her operative leg is painful, and she barely moves. During her bath, the nurse notes a shallow, open, reddened area 2 inches in diameter on her sacral area and a large tender purple area with intact skin on the heel of her right foot.

1. Why did these areas develop?

   _____

   _____

   _____

   _____

2. To plan Mrs. Miller's care, how would you stage these lesions?

   _____

   _____

3. The surgeon is notified of these areas and orders turning every 2 hours, elevation of the right foot, and a special pressure-reducing bed. What is the benefit and effectiveness of each of these ordered interventions?

   _____

   _____

   _____

   _____

   _____

   _____

REVIEW QUESTIONS—CONTENT REVIEW

Choose the best answer unless directed otherwise.

1. Which of the following activities creates a mechanical force that can lead to the formation of a pressure injury?
   1. Massaging nonreddened areas
   2. Whirlpool baths
   3. Pulling a patient up in bed
   4. Range-of-motion exercises

2. Which of the following dressings should a nurse choose for a deep pressure injury that has purulent drainage?
   1. Sterile gauze
   2. Transparent film (OpSite)
   3. Hydrocolloid (DuoDERM)
   4. Occlusive

REVIEW QUESTIONS—TEST PREPARATION

Choose the best answer unless directed otherwise.

3. A nurse is caring for a nursing home resident with a red, pruritic skin rash. The patient is confused and scratches the rash, which results in broken skin. Which interventions will help the rash heal? **Select all that apply.**
   1. Pat the skin dry after bathing.
   2. Leave topical agent as ordered at the bedside so the patient can apply when itching is severe.
   3. Place a transparent dressing on the rash to prevent scratching.
   4. Place gloves or mitts on the patient.
   5. Keep the patient's fingernails short.
   6. Place wrist restraints on the patient during the night.

4. A patient has a wound that is draining moderate blood-tinged clear fluid. Which of the following would be an appropriate description of this drainage for the nurse to document?
   1. Purulent drainage
   2. Serosanguineous drainage
   3. Copious drainage
   4. Serous drainage

5. The nurse is providing care for a patient with a noninfected stage 3 pressure injury. Which of the following actions is most appropriate for cleaning the wound?
   1. Flushing the wound with pressure of 45 pounds per square inch
   2. Gentle flushing with a needleless 30-milliliter syringe
   3. Gentle scrubbing with gauze and normal saline
   4. Flushing with a 30-milliliter syringe with an 18-gauge needle

6. A 62-year-old patient is admitted to the hospital with a lesion on the face that is a small, pearly papule. It has a rolled, waxy edge with crusting and ulceration. Which action by the nurse is best?
   1. Notify the physician.
   2. Clean the lesion.
   3. Place a gauze dressing on the lesion.
   4. Place an occlusive dressing on the lesion.

7. Place the wounds in correct order from stage 1 to stage 4.
   1. Skin appears abraded.
   2. Skin is red, intact, and nonblanchable.
   3. Full-thickness skin is lost; muscle and bone are showing.
   4. Full-thickness skin is lost; no muscle or bone involvement.

8. A 92-year-old patient is admitted from a nursing home to the hospital for a colon resection. Four days postoperatively, the patient reports that the perineum is sore. It is reddened and has whitish discharge. The patient has been on three intravenous antibiotics. Which of the following problems does the nurse suspect?
   1. Candidiasis
   2. Psoriasis
   3. Herpes zoster
   4. Contact dermatitis

9. The nurse recognizes that which of the following individuals should be evaluated for a specialty bed that provides a pressure-relieving surface?
   1. A 46-year-old with scoliosis who has a urinary tract infection
   2. A 94-year-old with a Braden score of 15 and left arm weakness from a cardiovascular accident
   3. An 88-year-old with foot drop who has a Foley catheter
   4. A 15-year-old with a Braden score of 9 who experiences pain with turning

CHAPTER 55
Nursing Care of Patients With Burns

Name: _____

Date: _____

Course: _____

Instructor: _____

AUDIO CASE STUDY

Listen to the audio case study available on Davis Edge and then answer the following questions.

Peyton and Burns

1. What do partial-thickness burns, superficial and deep, look like? Full-thickness?

_____

_____

_____

_____

_____

2. Which types of burns are most painful?

_____

_____

_____

_____

3. Why was Peyton at risk for fluid loss? How did Chris monitor Peyton's fluid status?

_____

_____

_____

_____

_____

_____

_____

_____

_____

4. Why did Peyton need extra caloric intake?

_____

_____

_____

_____

_____

VOCABULARY

Match each phrase with the type of burn or burn term.

1. _____ Leathery skin, usually painless
2. _____ Pink to red moist skin; blisters may be present
3. _____ The growth of skin over a wound
4. _____ Removal of a slough or scab formed on skin and underlying tissue of severely burned skin
5. _____ Epidermis and dermis involved, pain from exposed nerve endings
6. _____ Hard scab or dry crust from necrotic tissue

1. Debridement
2. Eschar
3. Epithelialization
4. Superficial partial-thickness burn
5. Partial-thickness deep burn
6. Full-thickness burn

CRITICAL THINKING

Read the following case study and answer the questions.

Mr. Patel is a 45-year-old patient in a burn unit. He was admitted with a 20% electrical burn over his right arm, right shoulder, right leg, and right foot. The entry wound is on his right shoulder, and the exit wound is on his right foot. When you check on him at the beginning of your shift, you find his right radial pulse is diminished and his right forearm has a small spot that is beginning to change color to a whitish gray.

1. What might be causing his change in circulation?

_____

_____

_____

_____

_____

2. What additional data should you collect? _____

_____

_____

_____

_____

3. What interventions are important to perform right away?

_____

_____

_____

_____

REVIEW QUESTIONS—CONTENT REVIEW

Choose the best answer unless directed otherwise.

1. Which cause of or type of burn is commonly associated with an inhalation injury?
   1. Electrical
   2. Flame
   3. Scald
   4. Contact

2. Which type of burn is caused by a hot liquid?
   1. Radiation
   2. Contact
   3. Scald
   4. Chemical

REVIEW QUESTIONS—TEST PREPARATION

Choose the best answer unless directed otherwise.

3. During morning report, a nurse is assigned a patient who is in stage 3 burn care. What care can the nurse anticipate providing during the shift?
   1. Dressing changes
   2. Debridement
   3. Pain management
   4. Exercises

4. A patient is brought to the emergency department with burns over 40% of the body from an apartment fire. Which assessment should take priority?
   1. Burn depth
   2. Percent of body surface burned
   3. Respiratory status
   4. Circulatory status

5. A home health care nurse visits an 82-year-old patient. On entering the home, the nurse finds that the patient has just dropped a pot of boiling water on both legs. What action should the nurse take first?
   1. Call 911.
   2. Remove the clothing from the affected area.
   3. Place ice on the affected area.
   4. Assess the extent of the burn.

6. A patient has a burn encircling the left thigh from a motorcycle accident. When the nurse enters the room during rounds, the patient appears very anxious and reports a funny feeling in the left foot. What should the nurse do first?
   1. Check circulatory status in the foot and report changes.
   2. Explain that some numbness and tingling in the affected extremity are normal following a burn.
   3. Check the burn dressing for an increase in drainage.
   4. Determine the cause of the patient's anxiety.

7. A homebound patient is receiving intravenous antibiotics for an infected burn site. Instructions are to use gravity to infuse 100 mL over 1 hour. How many drops per minute should the nurse administer if the tubing has a drip factor of 15? _____

8. A nurse is providing care for a patient with burns across 30% of the body. Which of the following observations would cause the nurse to contact the registered nurse or physician?
   1. Urinary output is 50 mL in the past 2 hours.
   2. Patient reports pain of 6/10; oral narcotic is due in 10 minutes.
   3. Respiratory rate is 20, and oxygen saturation is 94%.
   4. Blood sugar is 175 mg/dL.

9. While caring for a 28-year-old patient newly admitted for burns received in a household fire, the nurse would be most concerned by which of the following?
   1. Hematocrit is 48%.
   2. Blood pressure is 92/40 mm Hg.
   3. Pulse is 96 beats per minute.
   4. Respiratory rate is 22 per minute.

CHAPTER 56
Mental Health Function, Assessment, and Therapeutic Measures

Name: _____
Date: _____
Course: _____
Instructor: _____

AUDIO CASE STUDY

Bonnie: Ego Defense Mechanisms and Therapeutic Communication Techniques

Listen to the audio case study available on Davis Edge and then answer the following questions.

1. Bonnie yelled at her kids because she was frustrated with her instructor. Which ego defense mechanism was she using? What are other ego defense mechanisms?

   _____
   _____
   _____
   _____
   _____
   _____

2. Bonnie gave her kids money for ice cream to make up for yelling. What ego defense mechanism is she using now?

   _____
   _____

3. What are some therapeutic communication techniques Bonnie used with her daughter?

   _____
   _____
   _____
   _____
   _____

VOCABULARY

Fill in the blanks with the correct terms.

1. _____ is the way one adapts to a stressor.

2. The ability to think rationally and process thoughts is referred to as _____ ability.

3. _____ is the use of medication to treat psychological disorders.

4. _____ therapy uses an electric current to stimulate neurotransmitters in severely depressed patients.

5. A therapeutic _____ is a structured environment that aids in treatment of mental health disorders.

6. Psychoanalytic therapy can help clarify meaning and therefore help the patient gain _____ into an event or feeling.

7. _____ is assessed by asking a patient questions such as "Where are you now?" and "What year is it?"

8. The outward expression of feelings is called _____.

DEFENSE MECHANISMS

Name the defense mechanism being used in each of the following statements.

1. A patient with cancer says, "I know if I take my vitamins, I'll be fine." _____

2. A student comes unprepared to class and says, "I woke up late because my instructor gave us so much work to do, and I had to stay up all night, and my kids are sick, and the car isn't working." _____

3. A man who always wanted to be a lawyer but was not accepted into law school says, "Lawyers are all crooked. I would never trust one." _____

4. A teen who didn't make the football team says, "I've decided to give up trying to play in sports. I'm much better at piano." _____

5. A woman who was raped says, "Why are you calling me to set up rape counseling? I was not raped, and I do not need counseling." _____

6. A man who is passed over for a promotion yells at his son for a minor mistake, "You messed up again. You never do anything right." _____

7. An adolescent says to his mother, "I got a C on my project because you told me to do it all wrong."

   _____

8. The woman who cheated on an examination turns in extra work and states, "Here is some extra work I did. I really want to learn this material." _____

9. A teen tells her date, "I'm sorry I can't go out tonight. I have to wash my hair." _____

10. The student nurse tells the instructor, "I don't think I can do that catheter. I am feeling sick to my stomach. I think I ate some bad food in the cafeteria." _____

CRITICAL THINKING

Read the following case study and answer the questions.

Mrs. Jewel is a 48-year-old woman admitted to the medical unit with cellulitis of her lower legs and diabetes mellitus. She has arthritis and morbid obesity. As you collect some initial data, you notice that her hair is dirty and unkempt, her clothes are dirty, and she has an unpleasant body odor. You also find that she does not appear to have a good understanding of her health or self-care needs. You decide to assess her mental status.

1. What factors related to Mrs. Jewel's appearance provide information about her mental status? How can you find out if this is unusual behavior for her?

   _____

   _____

   _____

   _____

   _____

   _____

   _____

   _____

   _____

   _____

2. Mrs. Jewel is alert. What questions can you ask to assess orientation? _____

_____

_____

_____

_____

_____

_____

3. How might you determine whether Mrs. Jewel's thought processes are intact?

_____

_____

_____

4. What questions can you ask to determine Mrs. Jewel's recent and remote memory?

_____

_____

_____

_____

5. How do you determine speech and ability to communicate?

_____

_____

_____

_____

6. You determine that Mrs. Jewel's affect is inappropriate. What does this mean?

_____

_____

_____

_____

7. How can you evaluate Mrs. Jewel's judgment? _____

_____

_____

_____

_____

_____

8. How can perception be assessed? _____

_____

_____

_____

_____

_____

_____

REVIEW QUESTIONS—CONTENT REVIEW

Choose the best answer unless directed otherwise.

1. Which behavior in a patient with a chronic physical illness alerts the nurse to possible mental health concerns?
   1. The patient prays for healing from illness.
   2. The patient reads self-help books to gain insight into problems.
   3. The patient uses meditation to cope with chronic illness.
   4. The patient does not have any close friends.

2. Which defense mechanism is being used by the person who always seems to blame others for personal problems?
   1. Denial
   2. Projection
   3. Rationalization
   4. Transference

3. An office worker has an argument with the boss and, on arriving home, yells at the spouse and children. Which defense mechanism is being displayed?
   1. Rationalization
   2. Denial
   3. Reaction formation
   4. Displacement

REVIEW QUESTIONS—TEST PREPARATION

Choose the best answer unless directed otherwise.

4. The nurse is providing care for a patient immediately following electroconvulsive therapy. Which of the following nursing actions is most appropriate?
   1. Restrain the patient's extremities.
   2. Monitor the patient closely until he or she is oriented.
   3. Discharge the patient to home with instructions to rest.
   4. Administer oxygen at 4 L per minute.

5. The nurse is collecting admission data on a new patient with a long health history. Which of the following life events is considered a stressor?
   1. Gallbladder surgery at age 46
   2. Divorce at age 50
   3. Loss of job at age 55
   4. Whatever the patient says is stressful

6. A patient is admitted to the hospital mental health unit for behavior changes. The patient asks why magnetic resonance imaging has been ordered. Which response by the nurse is best?
   1. "Magnetic resonance imaging can determine levels of important neurotransmitters, so the doctor will know how to treat your problem."
   2. "Magnetic resonance imaging is used to rule out physical problems that could be causing your symptoms."
   3. "Magnetic resonance imaging uses magnetic energy to treat certain psychiatric disorders."
   4. "Magnetic resonance imaging monitors electrical activity in the brain to help diagnose mental health problems."

7. A patient with panic disorder tells the nurse that she has a lot of job-related stress. Which response by the nurse is most therapeutic for this patient?
   1. "Can you identify some of the things in your job that are causing you to feel stressed?"
   2. "I'm really sorry you have so much job stress."
   3. "It is important to eliminate stressful situations so you can reduce your panic attacks."
   4. "You need to avoid stressful situations. It would be wise to start looking for another job."

8. A patient who quit drinking 4 months earlier is considering entering an inpatient alcohol rehabilitation program and asks for the nurse's opinion. Which response by the nurse is best?
   1. "That is an excellent idea. I will help you start the paperwork."
   2. "Why do you think you need a rehabilitation program?"
   3. "What do you think you should do?"
   4. "You have done so well to be alcohol-free for 4 months."

9. A nurse is caring for a 36-year-old developmentally delayed patient admitted to the hospital for pneumonia. The patient becomes upset when the dinner tray is late and cries "Mama" repeatedly. The patient's mother later says this is unusual behavior for the patient. Which of the following is the best explanation for this behavior?
   1. The patient is having a conversion reaction based on the hospitalization.
   2. The patient is likely having a side effect to a new medication.
   3. The patient is having symptoms of regression.
   4. The patient is repressing feelings about the illness.

10. A patient stands up during a morning community meeting and screams, "Get out of here right now! The demons are coming!" Which response by the nurse is best?
    1. "Why do you think the demons are coming?"
    2. "Yes, we should all leave right now."
    3. "If you have something to say, you must only say it when it is your turn to share."
    4. "I know you think the demons are coming, but there are no demons. You are safe here."

CHAPTER 57

Nursing Care of Patients With Mental Health Disorders

Name: _____
Date: _____
Course: _____
Instructor: _____

AUDIO CASE STUDY

Samantha and Bipolar Disorder

Listen to the audio case study available on Davis Edge and then answer the following questions.

1. What symptoms of depression did Samantha experience?

   _____

   _____

2. What symptoms of mania did she experience?

   _____

   _____

3. What was Samantha experiencing when she thought the television show was real?

   _____

   _____

4. What treatment did Samantha receive for bipolar disorder?

   _____

   _____

VOCABULARY

Fill in the blanks with the correct terms.

1. A patient with schizophrenia who is unable to speak is experiencing

   _____.

2. A situation in which family members exist to enable a substance abuser is called

   _____.

3. An irrational fear is called a/an _____.

4. A repetitive thought or urge is called a/an _____.

5. Manic depressive illness is more appropriately called _____

   depression.

6. _____ spectrum disorder is characterized by social deficits and

   restricted repetitive behaviors.

7. People with _____ cannot distinguish between their reality and

   society's reality.

8. Abrupt withdrawal from alcohol may cause symptoms called _____

   tremens.

9. _____ is the repeated compulsive use of a substance despite negative

   consequences.

10. _____ refers to the loss of ability to enjoy things that are usually

    pleasurable.

CRITICAL THINKING

Read the following case study and answer the questions.

You are caring for Mr. Joers, a 72-year-old man admitted to your surgical unit from a nursing home after he fell and broke his hip. He is scheduled for surgery this morning at 0800. During morning report, you learn that he has a history of Parkinson disease, schizophrenia, and anxiety but that he was oriented and appropriate during admission and throughout the night. When you enter his room to check his vital signs and complete his preoperative checklist, he has a wild look in his eyes and says, "Don't come near me! They told me what you're up to!"

1. What is your initial response to Mr. Joers?

   _____

   _____

   _____

   _____

   _____

   _____

   _____

   _____

2. What implications does his behavior have for surgery this morning? _____

   _____

   _____

   _____

   _____

   _____

3. What may have precipitated his worsening symptoms?

   _____

   _____

   _____

   _____

4. What actions do you need to take after your initial response to Mr. Joers? _____

_____

_____

_____

_____

_____

5. What safety concerns do you have? _____

_____

_____

_____

_____

_____

_____

REVIEW QUESTIONS—CONTENT REVIEW

Choose the best answer unless directed otherwise.

1. Which of the following responses to anxiety is a cause for concern?
   1. A student studies late into the night to prepare for a difficult examination.
   2. A woman takes deep breaths before going into the grocery store because shopping makes her nervous.
   3. A nurse has a glass of wine before a stressful night shift.
   4. A young man gets the opinions of several of his friends before asking a woman out.

2. Which of the following is the most effective treatment for alcoholism?
   1. Group support, such as Alcoholics Anonymous
   2. Drug therapy
   3. Electroconvulsive therapy
   4. Slowly reducing amount of alcohol consumption

REVIEW QUESTIONS—TEST PREPARATION

Choose the best answer unless directed otherwise.

3. A patient being treated with lorazepam (Ativan) during alcohol withdrawal becomes sleepy after the first two doses and then becomes difficult to arouse when the nurse attempts to give the third dose. Which of the following actions should the nurse take first?
   1. Hold the dose and notify the registered nurse or physician.
   2. Understand that tolerance will occur with benzodiazepines and give the drug.
   3. Get the patient up and have him walk with assistance until he is more alert.
   4. Administer an antidote.

4. A patient calls a nurse into the room and says, "Quick, Nurse, there is a dog in the corner. Please get him out. I am terrified of dogs." The nurse sees no dog in the corner. Which of the following responses is best?
   1. "You know we don't allow dogs in the hospital."
   2. "We have been through this before. You know full well that there is no dog in the corner."
   3. "I do not see a dog. Let's take a walk down to the snack room."
   4. "What kind of a dog is it? What makes you so scared of dogs?"

5. A patient is starting on lithium for bipolar disorder. Which of the following nutrients should the nurse teach about maintaining in the diet?
   1. Potassium
   2. Sodium
   3. Selenium
   4. Tyramine

6. Which of the following behaviors by a nurse may aggravate the behavior of a patient with schizophrenia?
   1. Providing written instructions on when to take medications
   2. Speaking in short, simple sentences
   3. Maintaining a structured environment
   4. Speaking quietly to other staff members when the patient is present

7. A patient has an order for carbamazepine (Tegretol) 150 mg twice daily by mouth for bipolar disorder. It is supplied as a suspension, 100 mg in 5 mL. How many milliliters should the nurse prepare? _____

8. Which statement by a patient with depression indicates that nursing interventions have been helpful?
   1. "His comment upset me, but I reminded myself that it really isn't true."
   2. "I feel so hopeless about everything, but I am glad you are a good listener."
   3. "I feel so much better now that I know how to control my boss's behavior."
   4. "I am really trying to understand why everyone is against me."

9. A patient is beginning treatment with paroxetine (Paxil) for unipolar depression but after 10 days is still withdrawn and unable to participate in therapy. Which action by the nurse is best?
   1. Contact the ordering physician for an increase in the dose.
   2. Contact the ordering physician for an alternative antidepressant.
   3. Continue to support the patient while waiting for symptoms to subside.
   4. Encourage the patient to include St. John's wort, an herbal supplement, in the treatment regimen.

10. The nurse is providing care for a 28-year-old patient admitted for a cardiac arrhythmia. The patient is extremely thin. For what additional signs of anorexia nervosa should the nurse assess? **Select all that apply.**
    1. Distorted body image
    2. Electrolyte imbalances
    3. Dry skin
    4. Hyperthermia
    5. Hypotension